KU-467-594

Musculoskeletal Imaging Cases

Mark W. Anderson
Professor of Radiology and Orthopaedic Surgery
Department of Radiology and Medical Imaging
University of Virginia Health System
Charlottesville, Virginia

Stacy E. Smith
Chief and Barbara N. Weissman Distinguished Chair
Division of Musculoskeletal Imaging and Intervention
Department of Radiology
Brigham and Women's Hospital, Harvard Medical School
Boston, Massachusetts

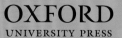

OXFORD
UNIVERSITY PRESS

OXFORD
UNIVERSITY PRESS

Oxford University Press is a department of the University of Oxford.
It furthers the University's objective of excellence in research, scholarship,
and education by publishing worldwide.

Oxford   New York
Auckland   Cape Town   Dar es Salaam   Hong Kong   Karachi
Kuala Lumpur   Madrid   Melbourne   Mexico City   Nairobi
New Delhi   Shanghai   Taipei   Toronto

With offices in
Argentina   Austria   Brazil   Chile   Czech Republic   France   Greece
Guatemala   Hungary   Italy   Japan   Poland   Portugal   Singapore
South Korea   Switzerland   Thailand   Turkey   Ukraine   Vietnam

Oxford is a registered trademark of Oxford University Press in the UK
and certain other countries.

Published in the United States of America by
Oxford University Press
198 Madison Avenue, New York, NY 10016

© Oxford University Press 2014

All rights reserved. No part of this publication may be reproduced, stored in a
retrieval system, or transmitted, in any form or by any means, without the prior
permission in writing of Oxford University Press, or as expressly permitted by law,
by license, or under terms agreed with the appropriate reproduction rights organization.
Inquiries concerning reproduction outside the scope of the above should be sent to the
Rights Department, Oxford University Press, at the address above.

You must not circulate this work in any other form
and you must impose this same condition on any acquirer.

Library of Congress Cataloging-in-Publication Data
Anderson, Mark W., 1957–
Musculoskeletal imaging cases / Mark W. Anderson, Stacy E. Smith.
    p. ; cm.—(Cases in radiology)
Includes bibliographical references and index.
ISBN 978–0–19–539437–5 (alk. paper)
I. Smith, Stacy E.   II. Title.   III. Series: Cases in radiology.
[DNLM: 1. Musculoskeletal Diseases—radiography—Case Reports.   2. Musculoskeletal System—radiography—Case
Reports.   3. Diagnosis, Differential—Case Reports.   4. Diagnostic Imaging—Case Reports. WE 141]
616.7′07572—dc23
2012046074

This material is not intended to be, and should not be considered, a substitute for medical or other professional
advice. Treatment for the conditions described in this material is highly dependent on the individual
circumstances. And, while this material is designed to offer accurate information with respect to the subject
matter covered and to be current as of the time it was written, research and knowledge about medical and health
issues is constantly evolving and dose schedules for medications are being revised continually, with new side
effects recognized and accounted for regularly. Readers must therefore always check the product information
and clinical procedures with the most up-to-date published product information and data sheets provided by
the manufacturers and the most recent codes of conduct and safety regulation. The publisher and the authors
make no representations or warranties to readers, express or implied, as to the accuracy or completeness of this
material. Without limiting the foregoing, the publisher and the authors make no representations or warranties as
to the accuracy or efficacy of the drug dosages mentioned in the material. The authors and the publisher do not
accept, and expressly disclaim, any responsibility for any liability, loss or risk that may be claimed or incurred as a
consequence of the use and/or application of any of the contents of this material.

9 8 7 6 5 4 3 2 1
Printed in China on acid-free paper

For Amy, whose patience, love and grace have made life so rich and
my professional endeavors possible, and to Jane, William, Charles and
John who have always kept me from taking it all too seriously!

Mark W. Anderson

To Jeff and Natalya with all my heart—I love you!!
And to all the trainees that I have had the pleasure of
working with—you make this all worthwhile!

Stacy E. Smith

Acknowledgments

I would like to thank my current colleagues in the Division of Musculoskeletal Imaging and Intervention, Brigham and Women's Hospital (BWH), Harvard Medical School in Boston (Piran Aliabadi, Barbara Weissman, Roger Han, Glenn Gaviola, Nehal Shah, and Kirstin Small) as well as our wonderful BWH MSK radiology fellows and residents for their assistance in finding great cases and sharing their enthusiasm for teaching and learning. In particular, I would like to thank Dr. Roger Han for his diligence in keeping and sharing such a great teaching file and providing some of the cases in this book as well as Dr. Kirstin Small for the great case of diffuse metabolic bone disease. I would also like to thank my former MSK colleagues, friends, and mentors (Chuck Resnik, Michael Mulligan, Nabile Safdar and Mark Murphey) and the great MSK radiology fellows, residents and medical students at the University of Maryland who provided such great support during my early faculty years in academic radiology and taught me that Academic Radiology isn't just a job but a great continuum of learning and sharing.

Mark W. Anderson

I would like to thank my mentors over the years who supported and encouraged me along my often circuitous route in academic medicine. From John McGahan and Adam Greenspan at the University of California at Davis to Clyde Helms, Phoebe Kaplan and Robert Dussault who gave me my start in MSK imaging and taught me what it meant to think like an MSK imager! And finally to Ted Keats who taught me the value of understanding how varied "normal" can be, and who showed me that learning and curiosity are tremendously effective at keeping you young, no matter what your chronologic age! And finally, a special thanks to all the residents and fellows who have listened, encouraged, challenged, and supported me over the years, while never knowing that I was the one fortunate enough to learn so much from them!

Stacy E. Smith

The Publisher thanks the following for their time and advice:

Mark W. Anderson, University of Virginia
Sanjeev Bhalla, Mallinckrodt Institute of Radiology, Washington University
Michael Bruno, Penn State Hershey Medical Center
Melissa Rosado de Christenson, St. Luke's Hospital of Kansas City
Rihan Khan, University of Arizona
Angela Levy, Georgetown University
Alexander Mamourian, University of Pennsylvania
Stacy E. Smith, Brigham and Women's Hospital, Harvard Medical School

Preface

Learning musculoskeletal (MSK) imaging should be fun. We both learned from great mentors through day to day work at the viewbox, case conference and, yes, even those things called books. During our time in academic radiology we have observed that the most effective means for learning seem to shift with each new generation. Today's radiology trainees might be best described as being a part of the the "tablet" or "technological gadget" generation and we have noted that the most productive learning is often through short case studies with pertinent images and simple but memorable points rather than an exhaustive text with many more words than images. We have tried to provide just that by including a wide variety of MSK pathology illustrated with multiple imaging modalities and explained with just enough text to cover the most important points about each.

We hope as you work through these cases that you'll begin to understand why we're so passionate about our chosen field, and that you'll gain some valuable pearls regarding MSK imaging, whether you are a radiology resident or fellow, a medical student or a radiologist in private practice who wants to brush up on your skills in this area. It has been a great experience to work together on this project and we hope you find that the time you spend going through this collection of great cases has been well spent!

Stacy E. Smith and Mark W. Anderson
Boston, Massachusetts and Charlottesville, Virginia

Contents

Part I

Arthritis

History

▶ Polyarthralgias

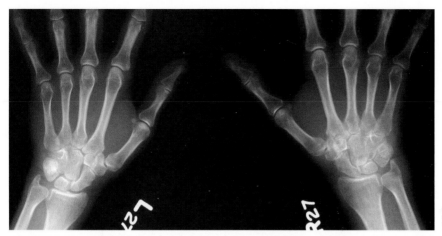

Figure 1.1

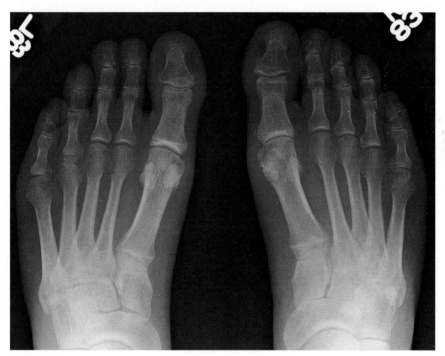

Figure 1.2

Case 1 Rheumatoid arthritis

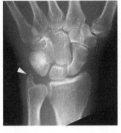
Figure 1.3

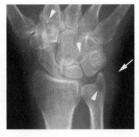
Figure 1.4

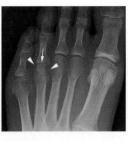
Figure 1.5

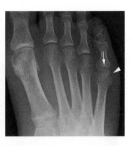
Figure 1.6

Findings

Figures 1.3 and 1.4 AP radiographs of the wrists (coned-down views from Fig. 1.1 on previous page) demonstrate scattered lucent erosions (*arrowheads*), most prominent in the right wrist, as well as fusiform soft tissue thickening along the ulnar aspect of the right wrist in the region of the extensor carpi ulnaris tendon (*arrow* in Fig. 1.4).

Figures 1.5 and 1.6 AP radiographs of the feet (coned-down views from Fig. 1.2 on previous page) reveal additional marginal erosions of the metatarsal heads (*arrowheads*) as well as uniform narrowing of the affected joints (*arrows*).

Differential Diagnosis

Seronegative spondyloarthropathies ("rheumatoid variants") such as psoriasis or reactive arthritis.

Teaching Points

▶ Rheumatoid arthritis is an inflammatory polyarthritis that most commonly affects women and may result in extensive articular deformities if untreated.
▶ In the hands and wrists, it tends to involve the carpal and metacarpophalangeal joints and often demonstrates a relatively symmetric distribution, although this is not always the case, as illustrated in this patient. Erosions of the ulnar styloid are also common. In the feet, the metatarsophalangeal joints are commonly affected.
▶ Classic radiographic findings include the following:
  ▪ Periarticular osteopenia (related to soft tissue hyperemia)
  ▪ Sharply defined, nonproliferative marginal erosions without sclerotic borders
  ▪ Uniform joint space narrowing (related to chondrolytic enzymes)
  ▪ "Boutonière" and "swan neck" deformities of the fingers (late)

Management

Nonsteroidal anti-inflammatory medications and/or corticosteroids in more mild cases. With more severe disease, disease-modifying antirheumatic drugs (DMARDs) may be used.

Further Readings

Jacobson JA, Girish G, Jiang Y, Resnick D. Radiographic evaluation of arthritis: inflammatory conditions. *Radiology* 2008;*248*:378–389.

History

► Wrist pain

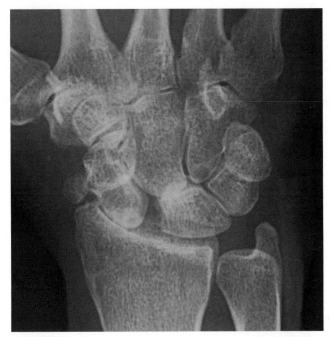

Figure 2.1

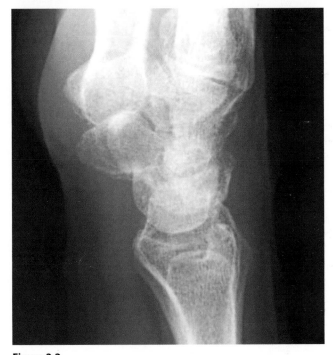

Figure 2.2

Case 2 SLAC (scapholunate advanced collapse) wrist

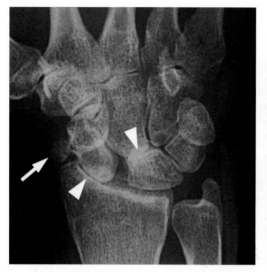 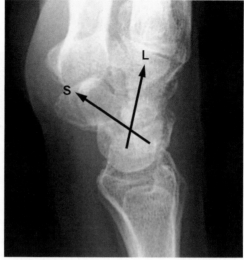

Figure 2.3   **Figure 2.4**

Findings

Figure 2.3, PA radiograph of the wrist, demonstrates widening of the scapholunate interval (scapholunate dissociation) and severe cartilage loss at the capitate–lunate and radioscaphoid joints (*arrowheads*). This constellation of findings is compatible with a SLAC wrist. Note also the old radial styloid fracture fragment (*arrow*). Figure 2.4, lateral radiograph, demonstrates the dorsal intercalated segmental instability (DISI) pattern commonly associated with a SLAC wrist. A DISI deformity is diagnosed when the angle formed by the axes of the scaphoid (*S*) and lunate (*L*) is greater than 60 degrees.

Differential Diagnosis

None

Teaching Points

▶ Disruption of the scapholunate ligament results in scapholunate dissociation with widening of the scapholunate interval and abnormal biomechanics in the proximal carpal row. Over time, the abnormal kinetics result in proximal migration of the capitate with progressive cartilage loss at the capitate–lunate joint as well as additional loss of cartilage at the radioscaphoid joint, as in this case.
▶ Common etiologies for a SLAC wrist include trauma, rheumatoid arthritis, and calcium pyrophosphate dihydrate crystal deposition disease (CPPD).
▶ Given the old fracture fragment adjacent to the radial styloid, trauma is the most likely etiology in this case.

Management

Surgical options include a proximal row carpectomy or wrist fusion.

Further Readings

Stabler A, Heuck A, Reiser M. Imaging of the hand: degeneration, impingement and overuse. *Eur J Radiol* 1997;25:118–128.

History

► Chronic neck pain

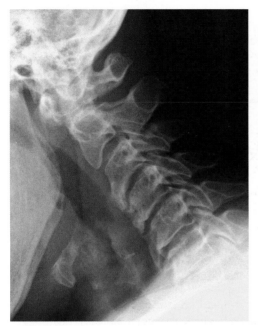

Figure 3.1

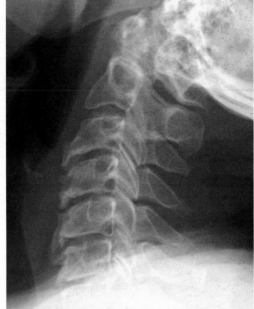

Figure 3.2

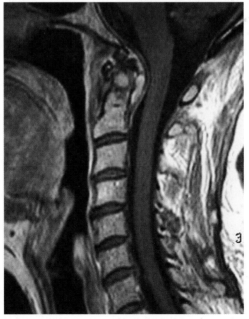

Figure 3.3

Case 3   Rheumatoid arthritis with atlantoaxial instability

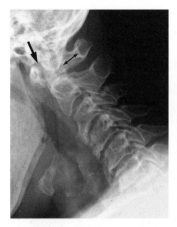

Figure 3.4

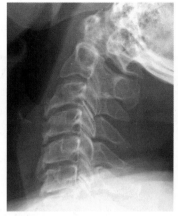

Figure 3.5

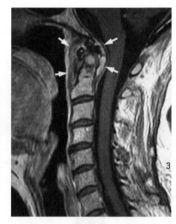

Figure 3.6

Findings

Figure 3.4, lateral view of the cervical spine in flexion, and Fig. 3.5, in extension, demonstrate mild widening of the predental space (*large arrow*) that corrects with extension, indicating atlantoaxial instability. (*Double-headed arrow* indicates the posterior atlantodental interval—see Teaching Points below.)

Figure 3.6, sagittal T1-weighted image of the cervical spine after intravenous gadolinium administration, reveals extensive enhancing tissue around the dens compatible with pannus related to the patient's rheumatoid arthritis (*arrows*).

Differential Diagnosis

Calcium pyrophosphate dihydrate crystal deposition disease (CPPD), gout, amyloid arthropathy

Teaching Points

► After the hands and feet, the cervical spine is the next most common site of involvement with rheumatoid arthritis, typically involving the synovial joints in the C1–2 region.
► Hypertrophied synovium (pannus) may weaken or rupture supporting ligaments (transverse, alar, apical), leading to atlantoaxial instability in up to 50% of patients. Cranial migration of the C2 vertebra (basilar invagination) may also occur.
► A predental space measuring more than 3 mm is suggestive of instability, but a posterior atlantodental interval (*double-headed arrow* in Fig. 3.4) measuring less than 14 mm is even more predictive of neurologic sequelae and is used by some as an indication for surgical stabilization.

Management

Medical treatment of rheumatoid arthritis. Surgical stabilization in cases of pronounced instability and/or neurologic deterioration.

Further Readings

Kim DH, Hilibrand AS. Rheumatoid arthritis in the cervical spine. *J Am Acad Orthop Surg* 2005;13:463–474.

History

▶ 50-year-old man with deformity, swelling, and pain bilateral hands and feet with history of skin disease

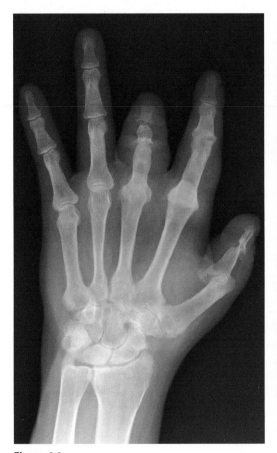

Figure 4.1

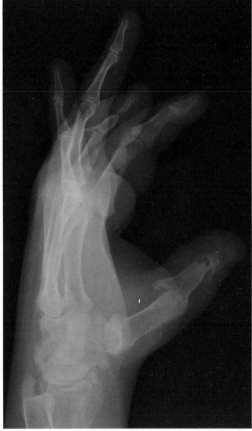

Figure 4.2

Case 4   Psoriatic arthritis

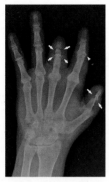 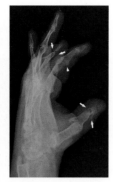

Figure 4.3   **Figure 4.4**

Findings

Figures 4.3 and 4.4 (AP and oblique hand radiographs) show fusiform soft tissue swelling of the third finger and, to a lesser degree, the second and first digits. There is an early marginal erosion with adjacent mild bone proliferation giving rise to a subtle "mouse ear" deformity at the second PIP joint (*white arrowhead*). More severe erosive disease and tuftal resorption give a "pencil-in-cup" appearance to the first IP joint, third PIP and DIP joints (*white arrows*). Subluxation is noted at multiple MCP joints. There is no evidence of osteoporosis.

Differential Diagnosis

Reactive arthritis, Erosive osteoarthritis, gout, infection

Teaching Points

▶ Marginal erosions characterize this disease, with the erosions of joints originating peripherally at bare areas and proceeding centrally to form early "mouse ear" and late severe "pencil-in-cup" deformities.

▶ Distal involvement predominates (unlike rheumatoid arthritis), with DIP involvement of the hands most common, followed by involvement of the feet, PIP, and MCP joints to a lesser degree. The sacroiliac joints and spine can also be involved.

▶ Typically there is an asymmetric bilateral distribution.

▶ Bone density is maintained, unlike other entities such as rheumatoid arthritis, as osteoporosis is not a prominent feature of psoriatic arthritis.

▶ Bone production is a feature of this disease, including bone proliferation adjacent to erosions, metaphyseal and diaphyseal periostitis, bone production at tendon and ligament insertion sites, and eventual ankylosis of joints in some severe cases.

▶ Severe cases may progress to arthritis mutilans.

▶ Soft tissue swelling is common, and predominant involvement of one digit is referred to as a "sausage digit."

▶ Skin disease is characteristic but may not always be present in conjunction with joint abnormalities.

Management

Early disease is treated conservatively with nonsteroidal anti-inflammatories, , corticosteroids, and physical therapy, with topical creams if skin disease is present. With more severe disease, disease-modifying anti-rheumatic drugs (DMARDS) may be used. Radiographic follow-up is often performed to monitor disease, especially during treatment and particularly if there is increased pain or swelling. Less than 10% of patients have complete remission.

Further Readings

Brower AC, Flemming DJ. Psoriatic arthritis. In *Arthritis in Black and White*, 2nd ed. Philadelphia, PA: Saunders, 1997:225–244.
Resnick D. *Diagnosis of bone and joint disorders*, 3rd ed. Vol. 2. Philadelphia, PA: W.B. Saunders, 1995:1075–1096.

History

▶ Pain and swelling

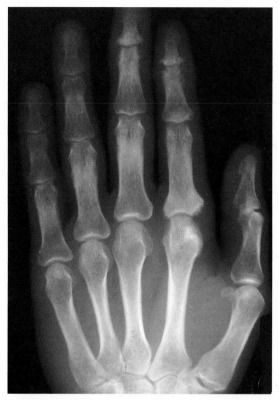

Figure 5.1

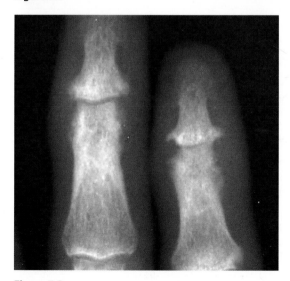

Figure 5.2

Case 5 Psoriatic arthritis

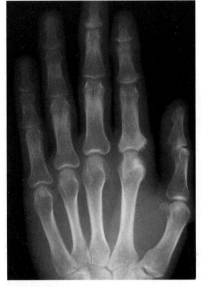

Figure 5.3

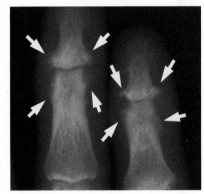

Figure 5.4

Findings

Figure 5.3, AP view of the hand, reveals marginal erosions and soft tissue swelling involving the DIP joints of the index and long fingers, shown to better advantage in the coned-down view (Fig. 5.4). Note also the associated areas of ill-defined ("fuzzy") bone proliferation (*arrows*).

Differential Diagnosis

Other seronegative spondyloarthropathies (reactive arthritis, ankylosing spondylitis, arthritis of inflammatory bowel disease)

Teaching Points

► The seronegative spondyloarthropathies include psoriatic arthritis, reactive arthritis ("Reiter's syndrome"), ankylosing spondylitis, and the arthritis associated with inflammatory bowel disease.
► All four tend to involve the sacroiliac joints and spine. Psoriatic and reactive types tend to also involve predominantly the hands and feet, while the others more commonly involve the central joints (e.g., hips).
► With psoriatic arthritis, marginal erosions typically involve the small joints of the hands and less commonly the feet. Reactive arthritis tends to involve the lower extremities more so than the upper.
► While the appearance may resemble rheumatoid arthritis, helpful differentiating features seen with psoriasis include asymmetric involvement of the distal (PIP and DIP) joints, a ray-like distribution of bone changes and soft tissue swelling ("sausage digit"), and especially the presence of ill-defined bone proliferation at the sites of involvement, as illustrated in this case.

Management

Nonsteroidal anti-inflammatory medications and/or corticosteroids are used in milder cases. With more severe disease, disease-modifying antirheumatic drugs (DMARDs) may be used.

Further Readings

Tan AL, McGonagle D. Psoriatic arthritis: correlation between imaging and pathology. *Joint Bone Spine* 2010;77:206–211.

History

► History of ankylosing spondylitis, s/p fall

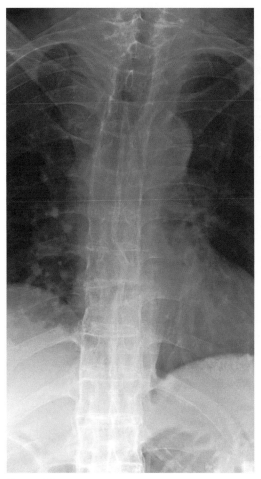

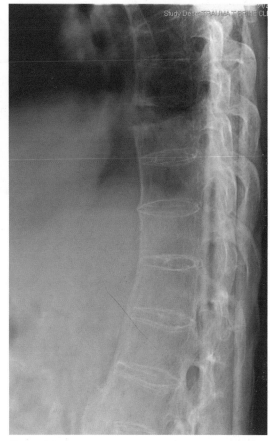

Figure 6.1 **Figure 6.2**

Case 6 Ankylosing spondylitis with fracture

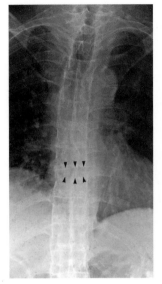

Figure 6.3

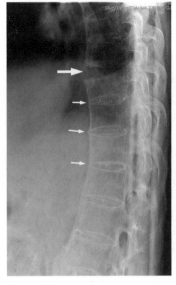

Figure 6.4

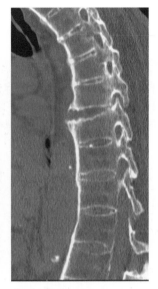

Figure 6.5

Findings

Figure 6.3, AP radiograph of the thoracic spine, demonstrates multilevel ankylosis with a subtle cleft-like lucency at the T8–9 level (*arrowheads*). Figure 6.4, lateral view, reveals the distracted fracture at that level to better advantage (large arrow). Additionally, thin marginal syndesmophytes, characteristic of ankylosing spondylitis, are better demonstrated at other levels (*small arrows*). Figure 6.5, sagittal reconstructed image from a CT scan of the thoracic spine, provides better delineation of the findings.

Differential Diagnosis

None

Teaching Points

▸ Spinal fractures can occur in patients with ankylosing spondylitis with even mild trauma owing to the rigidity of the fused spinal column. Fractures may extend through the ankylosed disk (as in this case) as well as through any part of the vertebral elements, and commonly involve all three columns of the spine.

▸ These injuries can be very difficult to detect with radiographs, especially in the mid to upper thoracic spine.

▸ CT is extremely useful for detecting these fractures and displaying their exact morphology. Likewise, MR imaging is useful for assessing associated cord and/or other soft tissue injuries.

▸ If not detected and treated, a fracture may go on to form a pseudoarthrosis (Andersson lesion).

Management

Surgical stabilization is usually required since these are typically very unstable fractures.

Further Readings

Wang Y-F, Teng MM-H, Chang C-Y, Wu H-T, Wang S-T. Imaging manifestations of spinal fractures in ankylosing spondylitis. *AJNR* 2005;*26*:2067–2076.

Westerveld LA, Verlaan JJ, Oner FC. Spinal fractures in patients with anklyosing spinal disorders: a systematic review of the literature on treatment, neurological status and complications. *Eur Spine J* 2009;*18*:145–156.

History

► Unknown

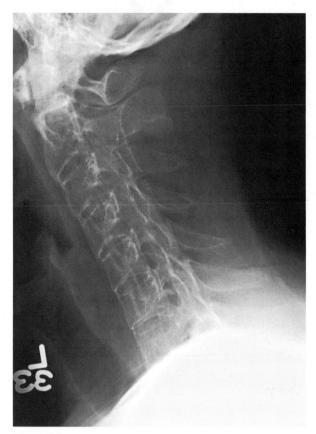

Figure 7.1

Case 7 Ankylosing spondylitis

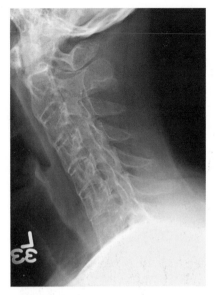

Figure 7.2

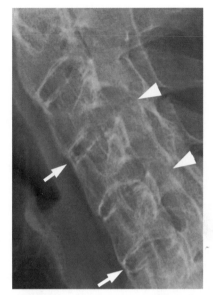

Figure 7.3

Findings

Figure 7.2, lateral radiograph of the cervical spine, demonstrates complete ankylosis of the spine. Figure 7.3, coned-down view, reveals the delicate, bridging marginal syndesmophytes that are characteristic of ankylosing spondylitis (*arrows*) as well as solid bony fusion of the facet joints (*arrowheads*).

Differential Diagnosis

Juvenile rheumatoid arthritis

Teaching Points

▶ The inflammatory spondyloarthropathies include ankylosing spondylitis, psoriatic arthritis, Reiter's syndrome (reactive arthritis), and the arthritis associated with inflammatory bowel disease. These typically affect the sacroiliac joints and result in varying degrees of ankylosis of the spine. Involvement of peripheral joints is less common.

▶ Anklyosing spondylitis often results in extensive ankylosis of the disk spaces, facet joints, and posterior elements, resulting in a "bamboo spine" appearance.

▶ The thin, marginal syndesmophytes present in this case are typical of patients with ankylosing spondylitis and inflammatory bowel disease, as opposed to the large, bulky, nonmarginal syndesmophytes seen with psoriatic arthritis and reactive arthritis.

▶ Longstanding juvenile rheumatoid arthritis may produce a similar appearance but can usually be differentiated clinically and often produces more vertebral deformities if associated with an onset in childhood.

Management

Physical therapy; nonsteroidal anti-inflammatory medications; corticosteroids; disease-modifying antirheumatic drugs (sulfasalazine); anti-TNF-alpha medication ("biologics").

Further Readings

Weber U, Kissling RO, Hodler J. Advances in musculoskeletal imaging and their clinical utility in the early diagnosis of spondyloarthritis. *Curr Rheumatol Rep* 2007;9:353–360.

History

► Low back pain

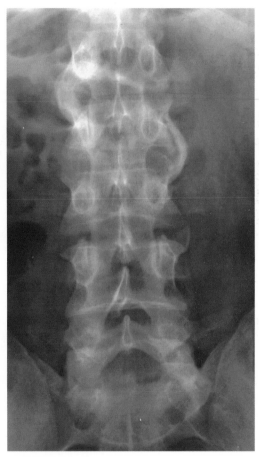

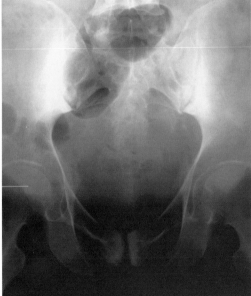

Figure 8.1

Figure 8.2

Case 8 Seronegative spondyloarthropathy: psoriatic arthritis

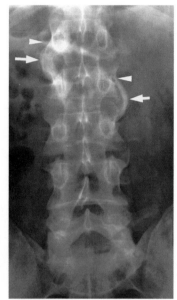

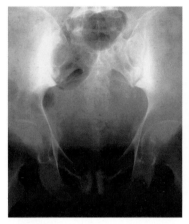

Figure 8.3   **Figure 8.4**

Findings

Figure 8.3, AP view of the pelvis, demonstrates irregularity and prominent marginal sclerosis along both sacroiliac joints compatible with sacroiliitis. Figure 8.4, AP view of the lumbar spine, reveals bulky, asymmetric nonmarginal syndesmophytes (*arrows*). Note how the syndesmophytes arise from the midvertebral bodies (*arrowheads*), unlike the marginal syndesmophytes of ankylosing spondylitis.

Differential Diagnosis

Osteophytes from degenerative disk disease; diffuse idiopathic skeletal hyperostosis (DISH)

Teaching Points

▶ The seronegative spondyloarthropathies include ankylosing spondylitis (AS), psoriasis, reactive arthritis (Reiter's syndrome), and enteropathic spondyloarthropathy (EPS) related to inflammatory bowel disease.

▶ All of these entities involve the sacroiliac joints and spine.

▶ AS and ES tend to produce symmetric sacroiliitis, while psoriasis and reactive arthritis tend to result in bilateral but asymmetric involvement; however, they can produce relatively symmetric findings, as in this case.

▶ Spinal involvement is markedly different between these entities, with AS and ES resulting in thin, symmetric marginal syndesmophytes and psoriasis and reactive arthritis producing thick, asymmetric paravertebral syndesmophytes that attach at the midvertebral body (nonmarginal).

Management

Nonsteroidal anti-inflammatory medications and/or corticosteroids in more mild cases. With more severe disease, disease-modifying antirheumatic drugs (DMARDs) may be used.

Further Readings

Tan AL, McGonagle D. Psoriatic arthritis: correlation between imaging and pathology. *Joint Bone Spine* 2010;*77*:206–211.

History

► Low back and foot pain

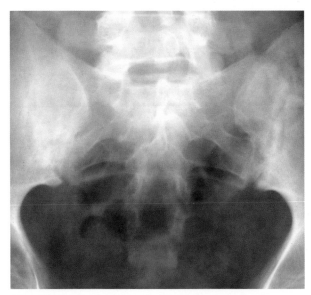

Figure 9.1

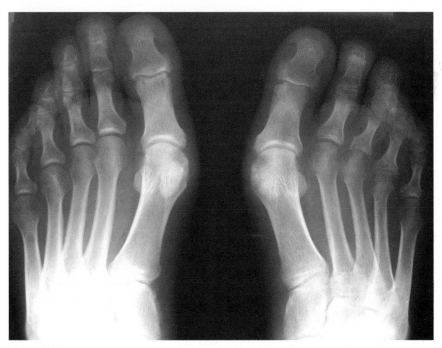

Figure 9.2

Case 9 Reactive arthritis (Reiter's Syndrome)

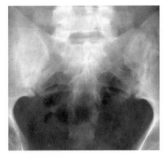

Figure 9.3

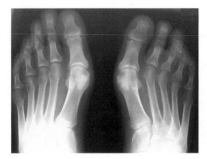

Figure 9.4

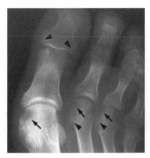

Figure 9.5

Findings

Figure 9.3, AP view of the sacroiliac joints, reveals ill-defined articular margins and periarticular sclerosis, right greater than left, compatible with sacroiliitis. Figure 9.4, AP view of both feet, demonstrates numerous, scattered marginal erosions that are better demonstrated in the coned-down view (*arrows* in Fig. 9.5). Note also the ill-defined areas of adjacent bone proliferation (*arrowheads*), as well as the uniform narrowing of the interphalangeal joint of the great toe.

Differential Diagnosis

Other seronegative spondyloarthropathies, especially psoriatic arthritis; rheumatoid arthritis (feet).

Teaching Points

▶ Reactive arthritis (also known as Reiter's syndrome) is one of the seronegative spondyloarthropathies, along with ankylosing spondylitis, psoriatic arthritis, and the arthritis related to inflammatory bowel disease.

▶ Classically, Reiter's syndrome consists of an arthritis, nongonococcal urethritis, and conjunctivitis.

▶ In most cases, this postinfectious arthritis tends to affect young men (male:female ratio = 3:1) and involves the joints of the lower extremity more commonly than those in the upper extremity.

▶ Involvement of the sacroiliac joints tends to be bilateral and asymmetric (indistinguishable from psoriatic arthritis). Within the appendicular joints, ill-defined, marginal erosions and adjacent areas of "fuzzy" bone proliferation are radiographic hallmarks of the disease.

▶ Other than the preponderance of lower extremity involvement, the findings are indistinguishable from those of psoriatic arthritis.

Management

The disease is usually self-limited, often within 2 to 6 months, but symptoms may require nonsteroidal anti-inflammatory medications and/or intra-articular corticosteroid injections. In more advanced cases, disease-modifying antirheumatic drugs (DMARDs) may be indicated.

Further Readings

Kim PS, Klausmeier TL, Orr DP. Reactive arthritis: a review. *J Adolescent Health* 2009;44:309–315.

History

▸ Low back pain

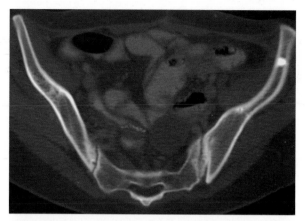

Figure 10.1

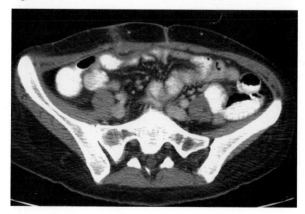

Figure 10.2

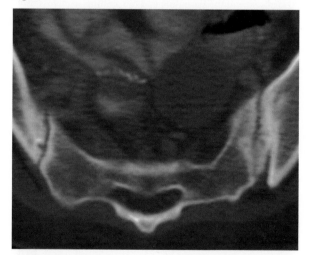

Figure 10.3

Case 10 Sacroiliitis/enteropathic spondyloarthropathy (Crohn's disease)

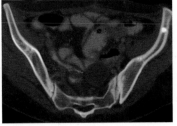
Figure 10.4

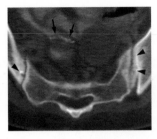
Figure 10.5

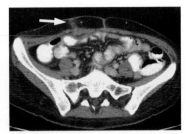
Figure 10.6

Findings

Figure 10.4 (and magnified image in Fig. 10.5), axial CT scan of the pelvis, reveals ill-defined articular margins, periarticular sclerosis, and small erosions (*arrowheads*) involving both sacroiliac joints, compatible with sacroiliitis. Note also the anastomitic surgical staples in the mid-pelvis (arrows). Figure 10.6, a scan at a higher level, demonstrates thickened loops of small bowel and a subcutaneous scar (*arrow*) from a prior ileostomy takedown in this patient with Crohn's disease. Note also absence of the ascending and descending segments of the colon related to a prior colectomy.

Differential Diagnosis

Other seronegative spondyloarthropathies (ankylosing spondylitis, psoriatic arthritis, reactive arthritis/Reiter's syndrome)

Teaching Points

▶ The seronegative spondyloarthropathies are a group of inflammatory disorders that include ankylosing spondylitis, psoriatic arthritis, reactive arthritis (Reiter's syndrome), and the arthritis related to inflammatory bowel disease (enteropathic spondyloarthropathy [EPS]).

▶ The most common bowel disorders associated with EPS are Crohn's disease and ulcerative colitis.

▶ Involvement of the sacroiliac joints tends to be bilateral and symmetric in this condition, indistinguishable from ankylosing spondylitis, although there may be some asymmetry in the degree of involvement. The classic findings in the spine (thin, marginal syndesmophytes, squaring of the vertebrae, etc.) are also similar in these two conditions.

▶ The combination of sacroiliitis and abnormal-appearing bowel, as in this case, may suggest the diagnosis of enteropathic spondyloarthropathy, but a specific diagnosis is usually made on clinical grounds.

Management

Medical therapies include standard drugs such as methotrexate and sulfasalazine, as well as newer agents such as pamidronate and tumor necrosis factor (TNF) blockers.

Further Readings

Gugliemlmi G, Scalzo G, Cascavilla A, Carotti M, Salaffi F, Grassi W. Imaging of the sacroiliac joint involvement in seronegative spondylarthropathies. *Clin Rheumatol* 2009;28:1007–1019.

Helliwell PS, Hickling P, Wright V. Do the radiological changes of classic ankylosing spondylitis differ from the changes found in the spondylitis associated with inflammatory bowel disease, psoriasis, and reactive arthritis? *Ann Rheum Dis* 1998;57:135–140.

History

► Painful hands

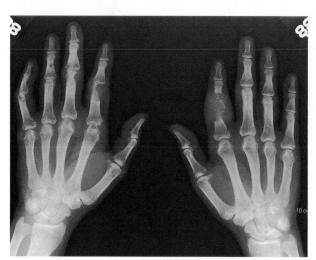

Figure 11.1

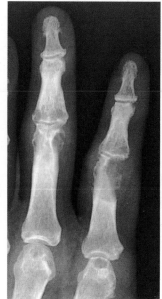

Figure 11.2

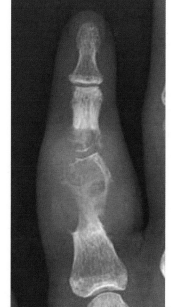

Figure 11.3

Case 11 Gout

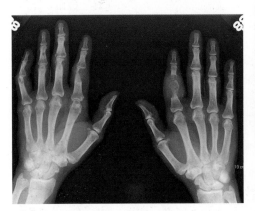

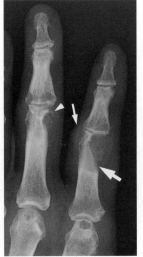

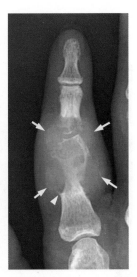

Figure 11.4

Figure 11.5

Figure 11.6

Findings

Figure 11.4, PA view of both hands, reveals extensive bilateral erosive changes involving the fingers with accompanying areas of nodular soft tissue prominence. Figures 11.5 and 11.6, coned-down views, demonstrate large para-articular erosions (*large arrow*), "overhanging edges" along some of the erosions (*arrowheads*) and high density within the areas of soft tissue prominence (*small arrows*).

Differential Diagnosis

Gout "mimickers": amyloidosis (especially in chronic dialysis patients); "cystic" rheumatoid arthritis; sarcoidosis; hyperlipidosis (rare); multicentric histiocytosis (rare)

Teaching Points

▶ Gouty arthritis is related to the deposition of urate crystals within joints and/or soft tissues (tophi). The resulting inflammatory changes produce pain and swelling, typically years before radiographic changes become evident.

▶ Classic radiographic findings include large erosions (may be marginal, para-articular, or intraosseous), often with characteristic "overhanging edges"; prominent nodular foci of localized soft tissue swelling that may demonstrate increased radiodensity related to urate crystals; and preservation of the articular cartilage until very late in the disease. Periarticular bone density is also usually preserved.

Management

Lifestyle and dietary changes; medications aimed at reducing serum uric acid levels

Further Readings

Perez-Ruiz F, Dalbeth N, Urresola A, deMiguel E, Schlesinger N. Imaging of gout: findings and utility. *Arthritis Research & Therapy* 2009;*11*:232–239.

History

▶ Great toe pain and swelling

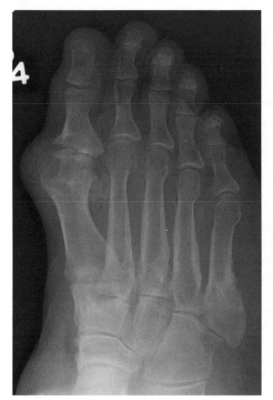

Figure 12.1

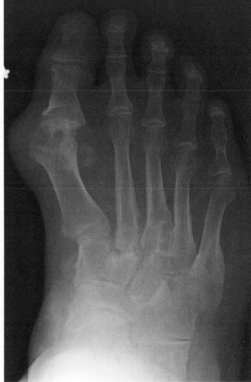

Figure 12.2

Case 12   Gout

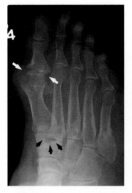
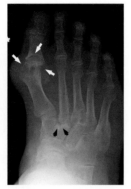

Figure 12.3   **Figure 12.4**

Findings

Figures 12.3 and 12.4 (AP and oblique radiographs): Large erosions with sclerotic borders and an overhanding edge of cortex most evident at the base of the first proximal phalanx are present at the medial and lateral sides of the first MTP joint (*white arrows*) with prominent medial soft tissue swelling and associated hallux valgus deformity. Erosion also noted at the second TMT articulation (*black arrows*). The first MTP joint space is relatively preserved. Other erosions are present near the TMT joints. Mineralization is normal and no soft tissue mineralization is present.

Differential Diagnosis

Psoriasis; infection; cystic "rheumatoid arthritis"

Teaching Points

► Gout arthropathy occurs secondary to deposition of monosodium urate crystals and has primary and secondary forms (the latter rarely demonstrates radiographic findings).
► Disease predominates in males (20:1).
► 65% of patients present with initial involvement of the first toe.
► Radiographic changes reflect the chronicity of the disease process.
► Radiographic manifestations include:
   1. Punched-out erosions with sclerotic borders ("mouse bite" appearance)
   2. Overhanging edge of cortex
   3. Joint space preservation
   4. Asymmetric polyarticular distribution (feet > ankles > knees > hands > elbow)
   5. Normal mineralization
   6. Tophi (soft tissue masses that may or may not calcify) in long standing disease.
► Spine and sacroiliac joint involvement may occur, but this is uncommon.

Management

MR may be useful in complex cases for further evaluation of joint disease and identification of calcific tophus adjacent to joint erosions. Image-guided aspiration of joint fluid is useful for crystal analysis in difficult cases. Dual energy CT has recently shown promise in differentiating gout from other arthropathies.

Further Readings

Brower AC, Flemming DJ. Gout. In *Arthritis in Black and White,* 2nd ed. Philadelphia: Saunders, 1997:325–343.
Yu J, Recht M, Dailiana T, Jurdi R. MR imaging of tophaceous gout. *AJR Am J Roentgenol* 1997;168:523–527.

History

► Knee pain

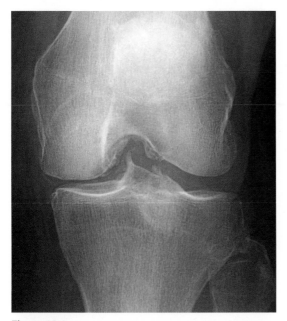

Figure 13.1

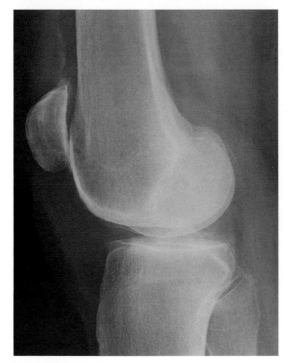

Figure 13.2

Case 13 Calcium pyrophosphate deposition disease (CPPD)

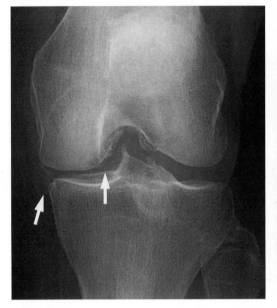

Figure 13.3

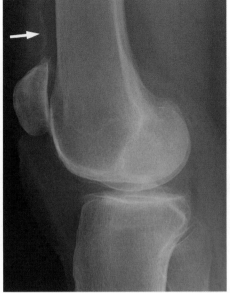

Figure 13.4

Findings

Figure 13.3 (AP radiograph) reveals narrowing of the medial joint compartment with some central spurring along the tibial spines. There are faint calcifications within the medial meniscus and articular cartilage (*arrows*). Figure 13.4 (lateral radiograph) shows severe narrowing of the patellofemoral joint compartment as well as curvilinear calcifications in the suprapatellar tissues (*arrow*).

Differential Diagnosis

Chondrocalcinosis (CPPD; hemochromatosis; hyperparathyroidism)

Teaching Points

▶ CPPD results in the deposition of calcium pyrophosphate crystals within joints and other soft tissues. Clinically, patients may experience acute, painful flares or more chronic symptoms.
▶ The disease may result in chondrocalcinosis (associated calcifications within hyaline articular cartilage and/or fibrocartilage such as the knee meniscus, glenoid labrum, etc.), a degenerative arthropathy, or both.
▶ Certain joints are more commonly involved with CPPD, such as the patellofemoral joint compartment of the knee and the radiocarpal joint of the wrist.

Management

Joint aspiration; nonsteroidal anti-inflammatories; corticosteroids (intra-articular or oral); colchicine (for acute flares)

Further Readings

Bencardino JT, Hassankhani A. Calcium pyrophosphate dihydrate crystal deposition disease. *Semin Musculoskelet Radiol* 2003;7:175–186.
Steinbach LS, Resnick D. Calcium pyrophosphate dehydrate crystal deposition disease: imaging perspectives. *Curr Probl Diagn Radiol* 2000;29:209–229.

History

▶ Chronic pain in hand and wrist

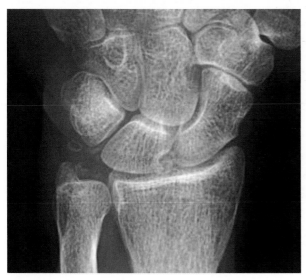

Figure 14.1

Case 14   Calcium pyrophosphate deposition disease (CPPD)

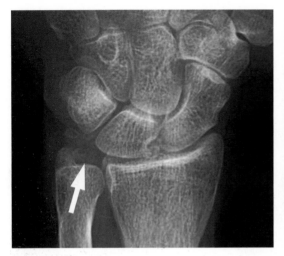

Figure 14.2

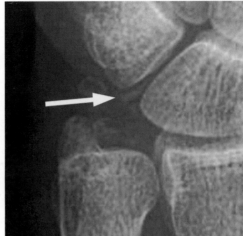

Figure 14.3

Findings

Figure 14.2 (AP radiograph of the wrist) reveals faint calcifications within the triangular fibrocartilage (*arrow*) compatible with chondrocalcinosis. Figure 14.3 (coned-down image) reveals additional calcification within the lunotriquetral ligament (*arrow*).

Differential Diagnosis

Chondrocalcinosis (calcium pyrophosphate deposition disease [CPPD]; hemochromatosis; hyperparathyroidism)

Teaching Points

▶ CPPD results in the deposition of calcium pyrophosphate crystals within joints and other soft tissues. Clinically, patients may experience acute, painful flares or more chronic symptoms.
▶ The disease may result in chondrocalcinosis (associated calcifications within hyaline articular cartilage and/or fibrocartilage such as the knee meniscus, glenoid labrum, etc.), a degenerative arthropathy, or both.
▶ Though the crystals may deposit within any tissues, common sites for chondrocalcinosis include the triangular fibrocartilage of the wrist, the symphysis pubis, and the menisci and/or articular cartilage of the knee.
▶ Certain joints are more commonly involved with CPPD, such as the patellofemoral joint compartment of the knee and the radiocarpal joint of the wrist.

Management

Joint aspiration; nonsteroidal anti-inflammatories; corticosteroids (intra-articular or oral); colchicine (for acute flares).

Further Readings

Bencardino JT, Hassankhani A. Calcium pyrophosphate dihydrate crystal deposition disease. *Semin Musculoskelet Radiol* 2003;7:175–186.
Steinbach LS, Resnick D. Calcium pyrophosphate dihydrate crystal deposition disease: imaging perspectives. *Curr Probl Diagn Radiol* 2000;29:209–229.

History

▶ 44-year-old woman with left hip femoral resurfacing prosthesis and left hip pain

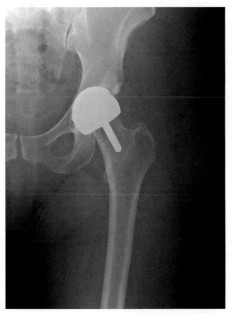

Figure 15.1

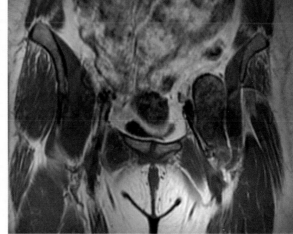

Figure 15.2

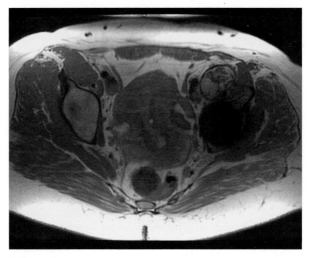

Figure 15.3

Case 15   Acute lymphocyte-dominated vasculitis-associated lesion (ALVAL)

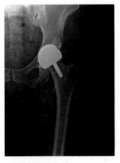

Figure 15.4

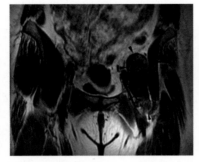

Figure 15.5

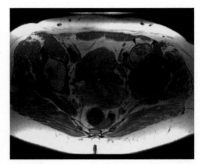

Figure 15.6

Findings

Figure 15.4 (AP radiograph left hip) shows a left femoral resurfacing component without foreign body, metallic debris, displacement, or abnormal lucency about the hardware. Figure 15.5 (coronal T1 MR pelvis) demonstrates a bilobed heterogeneous intermediate-signal collection within the left iliopsoas region (*black arrowheads*) with a thick peripheral low-signal rim. Figure 15.6 (axial PD MR pelvis) better demonstrates the well-defined low-signal-rimmed focal left iliopsoas collection (*black arrowheads*) with high-signal-intensity and low-signal-intensity central material characteristic of an ALVAL pseudotumor.

Differential Diagnosis

Rheumatoid arthritis; foreign body reaction; infection; mechanical loosening (metal or cement debris or particles more prevalent than in ALVAL)

Teaching Points

▸ Acute lymphocyte-dominated vasculitis-associated lesion (ALVAL) is a previously unrecognized complication of second-generation metal-on-metal (MOM) prostheses. It is thought to be caused by metal alloy ions (cobalt, chromium, molybdenum, or nickel) released by normal arthroplasty wear reacting with native proteins in the adjacent periprosthetic soft tissues, resulting in a type IV delayed hypersensitivity reaction.

▸ ALVAL is characterized by a dense perivascular inflammatory infiltrate, as in this case, and can lead to osteolysis and loosening of the prosthesis.

▸ Patients present with nonspecific symptoms or pain.

▸ Imaging is critical for identifying the potential "pseudotumor" that is the hallmark of this process. MR STIR sequences are preferable over fat-saturated sequences in patients with metal prostheses to avoid marked metallic artifact. Metal artifact reduction sequences and newer metal-specific sequences are useful in these cases.

Management

Intraoperative findings of chronic inflammation (ALVAL) require replacement of the prosthetic component surfaces.

Further Readings

Watters TS, Cardona DM, Menon KS, Vinson EN, Bolognesi MP, Dodd LG Aseptic lymphocyte dominated vasculitis associated lesion. A clinicopathologic review of an underrecognized cause of prosthetic failure *Am J Clin Pathol* 2010;*134*:886–893.

History

▶ Arthritis

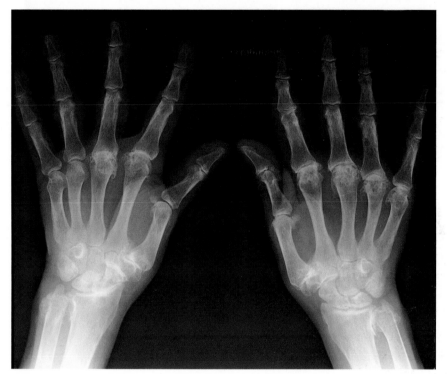

Figure 16.1

Case 16 Hemochromatosis

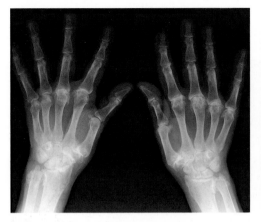

Figure 16.2

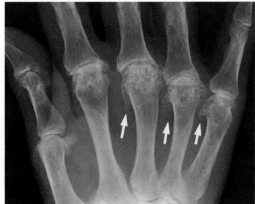

Figure 16.3

Findings

Figure 16.2 (PA view of the hands) reveals extensive, relatively symmetric arthritic changes that are most severe in the MCP joints. Figure 16.3 (coned-down view) shows severe, uniform cartilage loss in all of the MCP joints as well as large, hook-like osteophytes (*arrows*).

Differential Diagnosis

Calcium pyrophosphate dihydrate deposition disease (CPPD); osteoarthritis

Teaching Points

▶ Hemochromatosis is a disease that results in excess absorption and deposition of iron within the body. It affects both visceral organs as well as synovial joints.

▶ The disease can affect any joint, but is most commonly seen in the MCP joints, especially the second and third, a distribution that is identical to that of CPPD.

▶ Typical radiographic findings include severe, often uniform, cartilage loss with large osteophytes and rounded subchondral lucencies. Chondrocalcinosis is also present in approximately 30% of patients.

▶ The appearance is radiographically indistinguishable from CPPD, but a possible differentiating feature is that hemochromatosis often involves more joints, such as all of the MCP joints, as in this case.

▶ Ultimate diagnosis requires laboratory evidence of abnormal iron metabolism or even liver biopsy.

Management

Treatment involves removal of excess iron via phlebotomies and/or chelating agents.

Further Readings

Jager HJ, Mehring U-M, Gotz GF, et al. Radiological features of the visceral and skeletal involvement of hemochromatosis. *Eur Radiol* 1997;7:1199–1206.

History

▶ Pain with swallowing

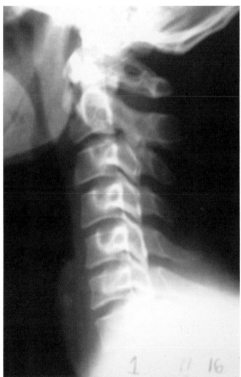

Figure 17.1

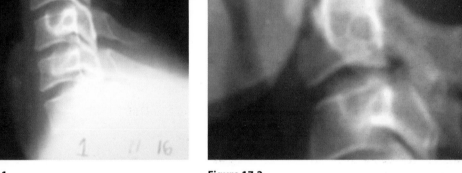

Figure 17.2

Case 17 Calcium hydroxyapatite deposition disease (HADD), longus colli muscle

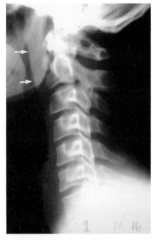

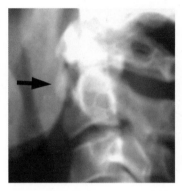

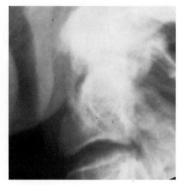

Figure 17.3   **Figure 17.4**   **Figure 17.5**

Findings

Figure 17.3 (lateral view of the cervical spine) demonstrates soft tissue swelling in the upper cervical region (*arrows*) as well as a smooth, ovoid calcific density anterior to the C2 vertebrae, better demonstrated on the coned-down view in Fig. 17.4 (*arrow*). Figure 17.5, a coned-down lateral view obtained 6 months later, shows resolution of these changes.

Differential Diagnosis

None

Teaching Points

▸ HADD, also known as calcific tendinitis, is a benign, self-limiting condition that most commonly affects the shoulders and hips.

▸ HADD involving the longus colli muscle, as in this case, results in acute retropharyngeal calcific tendinitis, a painful condition that can clinically mimic a prevertebral abscess or traumatic injury.

▸ Radiographic findings include prevertebral soft tissue swelling and focal, amorphous calcification at the C1-C3 level.

▸ Symptoms resolve spontaneously, often within just a few weeks. Follow-up imaging demonstrates resolution of the soft tissue abnormalities.

Management

Although this is a self-limited condition, symptomatic treatment may include nonsteroidal anti-inflammatory medications, analgesics, and, if needed, immobilization.

Further Readings

Chung T, Rebello R, Gooden EA. Retropharyngeal calcific tendinitis: case report and review of literature. *Emerg Radiol* 2005;*11*:375–380.

Park SY, Jin W, Lee SH, Park JS, Yang DM, Ryu N. Acute retropharyngeal calcific tendinitis: a case report with unusual location of calcification. *Skeletal Radiol* 2010;39:817–820.

History

▶ Left hip pain

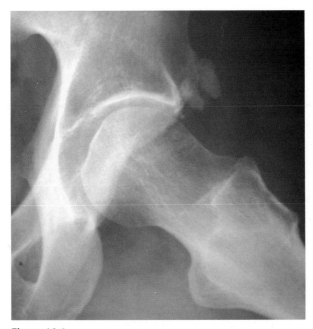

Figure 18.1

Case 18 Calcium hydroxyapatite deposition disease (HADD), left rectus femoris tendon

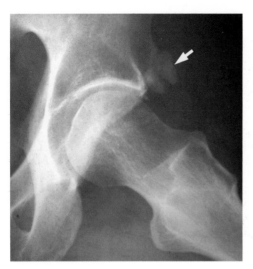

Figure 18.2

Findings

Figure 18.2 (frog-leg lateral view of the left hip) demonstrates a cluster of amorphous calcific densities (*arrow*) adjacent to the anterior inferior iliac spine at the site of the proximal rectus femoris tendon.

Differential Diagnosis

Other crystal deposition diseases (calcium pyrophosphate dihydrate disease [CPPD], gout), metabolic disorders (chronic renal disease, hypervitaminosis D, etc.), or collagen vascular diseases (dermatomyositis, systemic lupus erythematosus)

Teaching Points

▶ HADD results from the deposition of calcium crystals in the soft tissues, often in and around tendons, and is often referred to as "calcific tendinitis."

▶ It most commonly affects the shoulder (especially the supraspinatus tendon), with the hip, elbow, wrist, and knee being less commonly affected.

▶ Although this often results in recurrent painful episodes, it can be asymptomatic in many patients, and the deposits may spontaneously disappear.

▶ Although the sites of involvement are variable, the radiographic appearance of the deposits is fairly characteristic: one or more foci of amorphous calcification often with ill-defined margins (though they may appear quite discrete).

▶ Occasionally, erosion or even invasion of the adjacent bone may occur, potentially mimicking a surface neoplasm.

Management

Nonsteroidal anti-inflammatory medications; image-guided needle aspiration and steroid injection has also been shown to be effective in shortening the course of symptoms.

Further Readings

Siegal DS, Wu JS, Newman JS, Del Cura JL, Hochman MG. Calcific tendinitis: a pictorial review. *Can Assoc Radiol J* 2009;60:263–272.

History

▶ Knee pain

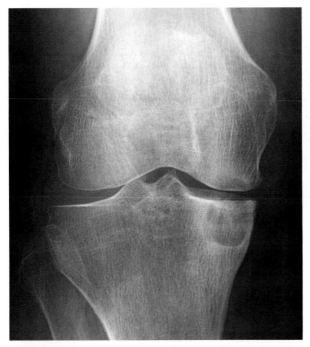

Figure 19.1

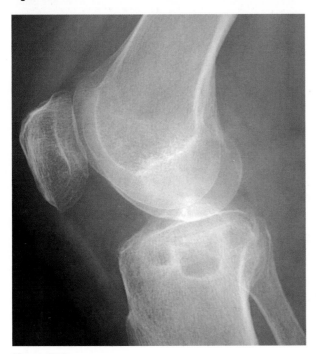

Figure 19.2

Case 19 Osteoarthritis with prominent subchondral cysts ("geodes")

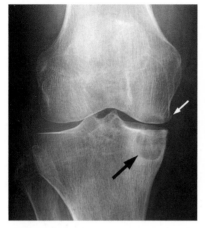

Figure 19.3

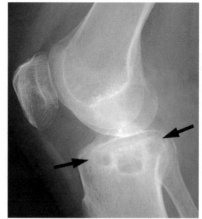

Figure 19.4

Findings

Figure 19.3 (frontal view of the knee) demonstrates medial joint space narrowing with an associated marginal osteophyte (*white arrow*) and a prominent, well-circumscribed rounded lucency in the proximal tibia compatible with a subchondral cyst (*black arrow*). Figure 19.4 (lateral view of the knee) demonstrates additional cysts within the proximal tibia (*arrows*).

Differential Diagnosis

None in this case, but in some patients a subchondral cyst may mimic other subarticular lesions, including giant cell tumor, Brodie's abscess, or chondroblastoma.

Teaching Points

▶ Subchondral cysts are seen in approximately 50% of patients with osteoarthritis. In the knee, their presence is associated with increased cartilage loss and a higher risk of joint replacement.

▶ Two mechanisms have been proposed regarding their etiology. The "synovial fluid intrusion" theory posits that they are secondary to areas of overlying full-thickness cartilage loss that allow synovial fluid to burrow into the subchondral bone. The "bone contusion" theory suggests that these develop at sites of bone injury and necrosis that are related to increased loading of the subchondral bone. Recent MR imaging studies have supported the latter theory by demonstrating a strong association between early subchondral foci of edema-like signal and subsequent cyst formation at those sites in patients with osteoarthritis. Similarly, there was no significant association between initial cartilage thickness and cyst development.

Management

Symptomatic treatment (nonsteroidal anti-inflammatories, intra-articular steroid or viscosupplement/hyaluronidase injections). Ultimately, joint replacement may be necessary.

Further Readings

Crema MD, Roemer FW, Zhu Y, et al. Subchondral cystlike lesions develop longitudinally in areas of bone marrow edema-like lesions in patients with or at risk for knee osteoarthritis: detection with MR imaging—the MOST study. *Radiology* 2010;256:855–862.

Tanamas SK, Wluka AE, Pelletier J-P, et al. The association between subchondral bone cysts and tibial cartilage volume and risk of joint replacement in people with knee osteoarthritis: a longitudinal study. *Arthritis Research & Therapy* 2010;12:R58.

History

▶ Chronic pain in hand and wrist

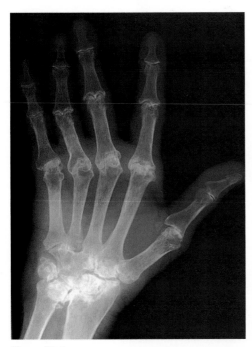

Figure 20.1

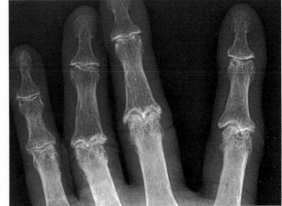

Figure 20.2

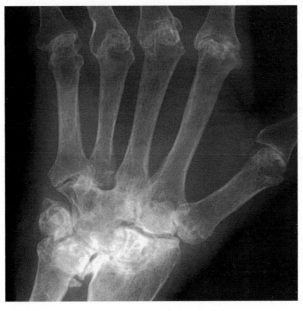

Figure 20.3

Case 20   Erosive osteoarthritis and coexistent rheumatoid arthritis

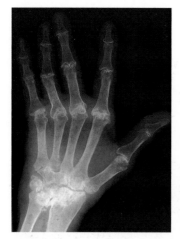

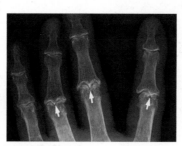

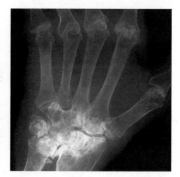

Figure 20.4   **Figure 20.5**   **Figure 20.6**

Findings

Figure 20.4 (AP radiograph of the hand) reveals extensive arthritic changes involving the joints of the hand and wrist. Figure 20.5 (coned-down view of the fingers) shows to better advantage the central erosions involving the PIP joints of the index, long, and ring fingers and associated osteophytes producing the typical "gull-wing" appearance of erosive osteoarthritis (*arrows*). Figure 20.6 (coned-down radiograph of the wrist) reveals severe pancarpal joint space narrowing and collapse as well as widespread erosions. Note also the severe, uniform narrowing of the MCP joints, associated erosions, and ulnar deviation at the third through fifth joints. These findings are compatible with rheumatoid arthritis.

Differential Diagnosis

Rheumatoid variants (psoriasis, Reiter's syndrome)

Teaching Points

▶ Erosive osteoarthritis produces typical findings in the interphalangeal joints of the fingers, most often in middle-aged to elderly women.

▶ The predominant findings are those of osteoarthritis: joint space narrowing, subchondral sclerosis, prominent periarticular osteophytes.

▶ The characteristic finding in this erosive variant is the additional finding of central "erosions," though some believe that these are actually areas of subchondral collapse. This combination of findings then results in the typical "gull-wing" appearance of the interphalangeal joints.

▶ In one study, 15% of patients with erosive osteoarthritis were found to have coexistent rheumatoid arthritis as seen in this case.

Management

Physical therapy; nonsteroidal anti-inflammatories; corticosteroids

Further Readings

Erlich GE. Inflammatory osteoarthritis—II: the superimposition of rheumatoid arthritis *J Chronic Dis* 1972;25:635–638.
Greenspan A. Erosive osteoarthritis. *Semin Musculoskelet Radiol* 2003;7:155–159.

History

► Routine chest radiograph

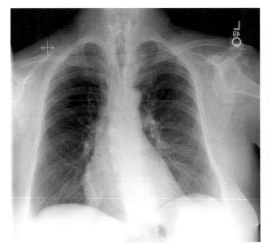

Figure 21.1

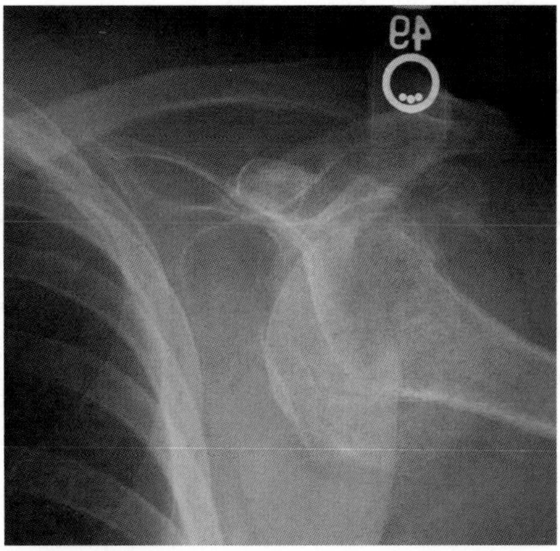

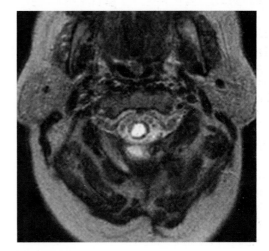

Figure 21.2

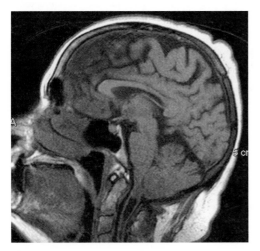

Figure 21.3

Figure 21.4

Case 21   Neuropathic arthropathy of the left shoulder secondary to a syrinx of the cervical spinal cord

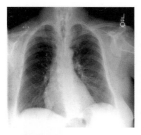

Figure 21.5

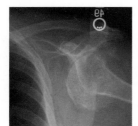

Figure 21.6

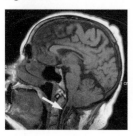

Figure 21.7

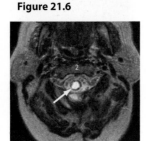

Figure 21.8

Findings

Figure 21.5 (PA view of the chest) and 21.6 (coned-down frontal view of the left shoulder) reveal dislocation and severe fragmentation of the left shoulder. In the absence of prior trauma or known dislocation, this is compatible with neuropathic arthropathy. Figure 21.7 (sagittal T1-weighted image of the head and neck) reveals a low-signal collection within the upper cervical spinal cord (*arrow*). Figure 21.8 (corresponding axial T2-weighted image) shows diffusely high signal within this cervical syrinx that nearly replaces the spinal cord at that level (*arrow*; 2 = C2 vertebra).

Differential Diagnosis

Prior trauma-related fracture-dislocation of the shoulder

Teaching Points

- ▸ Neuropathic arthropathy (also known as Charcot arthropathy) is secondary to a lack of sensation and proprioception leading to long-term damage to the structures of the involved joint.
- ▸ Radiographic findings are characteristic and typically consist of the "5 D's": increased density; bone destruction and disorganization, dislocation, and debris.
- ▸ This is most commonly encountered in the foot in diabetic patients. Other etiologies include spinal cord injury or syrinx, alcoholic neuropathy, leprosy, syphilis and congenital insensitivity to pain.
- ▸ Involvement of the shoulder is most often due to a syrinx in the cervical spinal cord, as in this case. Bilateral involvement may be seen.

Management

Palliative care; wound precautions (especially in a diabetic patient with foot involvement)

Further Readings

Hatzis N, Kaar TK, Wirth MA, Toro F, Rockwood CA Jr. Neuropathic arthropathy of the Shoulder. *J Bone Joint Surg Am* 1998;*80*:1314–1319.

Ruette P, Stuyck J, Debeer P. Neuropathic arthropathy of the shoulder and elbow associated with syringomyelia: a report of 3 cases. *Acta Orthop Belg* 2007;*73*:525–529.

History

▶ 27-year-old woman

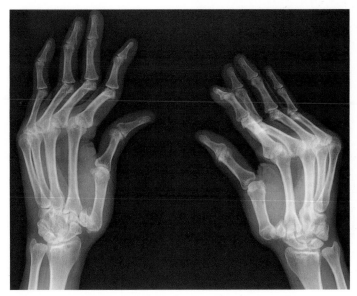

Figure 22.1

Case 22   Systemic lupus erythematosus (SLE; "Jaccoud's arthropathy")

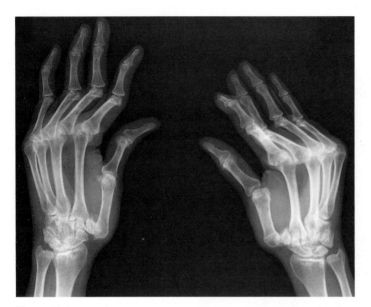

Figure 22.2

Findings

Figure 22.2 (PA view of the hands) reveals severe, bilateral deformities predominantly involving the MCP and interphalangeal joints without associated erosions.

Differential Diagnosis

Rheumatoid arthritis

Teaching Points

► While the majority of SLE patients have some degree of joint pain, only about 5% will develop a severe, deforming arthritis that is also known as "Jaccoud's arthropathy."

► The deformities tend to affect the MCP and PIP joints and are thought to result from ligamentous laxity and muscle imbalance, as opposed to the tissue destruction that produces similar deformities in patients with rheumatoid arthritis.

► While the changes resemble rheumatoid arthritis, the absence of erosions in SLE arthropathy is a discriminating feature.

► The presence of deformities and erosions in a patient with known SLE suggests the diagnosis of "rhupus," a condition that is thought to be a type of erosive SLE or, less likely, the coexistence of both SLE and rheumatoid arthritis.

Management

Depending on the severity of disease, treatment may involve nonsteroidal anti-inflammatory medications, corticosteroids, or more potent immunosuppressive drugs.

Further Readings

Fernandez A, Quintana G, Matteson EL, et al. Lupus arthropathy: historical evolution from deforming arthritis to rhupus. *Clin Rheumatol* 2004;23:523–526.

Ostendorf B, Scherer A, Specker C, Modder U, Schneider. Jaccoud's arthropathy in systemic lupus erythematosus: differentiation of deforming and erosive patterns by magnetic resonance imaging. *Arthritis Rheumatism* 2003;48:157–165.

History

▸ Bilateral hand pain and swelling with skin disease

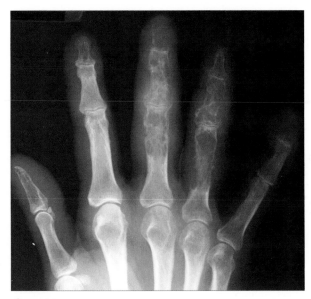

Figure 23.1

Case 23   Sarcoid

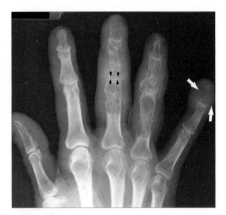

Figure 23.2

Findings

Figure 23.2 (Frontal radiograph of the fingers): Lacelike pattern of lucency and coarse trabeculae within the phalanges of the third and fourth digits, soft tissue swelling of the third and fourth digits and punched-out lytic lesion of the fifth DIP joint(*white arrows*).Preservation of joint spaces (*black arrowheads*) with no evidence of periostitis.

Differential Diagnosis

Enchondromatosis; sarcoidosis; hemangiomatosis; infection; psoriasis

Teaching Points

▶ Noncaseating granulomatous lesions are characteristic of sarcoidosis and underlie the lacelike bone appearance caused by the development of cystic areas with sclerotic rimmed scalloping and ossific deformity, with trabecular coarsening and eventual destruction of bone.
▶ The hands are predominately involved with the most common sites the middle and distal phalanges and then the proximal phalanges.
▶ Bone involvement occurs in about 5% of patients and is rare if there are no cutaneous findings (i.e., subcutaneous nodules).
▶ 80% of patients with bone involvement have abnormal chest radiographs.
▶ Periostitis, joint involvement (seen in only 10%), and soft tissue calcifications/phleboliths are NOT characteristics of this disease and help to differentiate it from psoriasis, infection, and tuberous sclerosis as well as enchondromatosis and Maffucci syndrome, respectively.
▶ Dactylitis is a rare complication. Acro-osteolysis has been reported as a nonspecific sign.

Management

Radiographic follow-up is the mainstay of evaluation for diagnosis and for evaluation during treatment, with MR imaging useful if there is severe progression of disease with increased pain or muscle symptoms, as the latter is more sensitive for detecting soft tissue abnormality. Glucocorticosteroids and methotrexate are modes of treatment. Imaging is recommended for evaluation of bone mineral density, as low bone mineral density and vitamin D/calcium balance disruption have been reported as potential complications.

Further Readings

Chew F. Radiology of the hands: review and self-assessment module. *AJR Am J Roentgenol* 2005;*184*:157–168.
Moore S, Tierstein A. Musculoskeletal sarcoidosis: Spectrum of MR imaging. *Radiographics* 2003;*23*:1389–1399.
Resnik D. *Diagnosis of bone and joint disorders*, 3rd ed., vol. 6. Philadelphia: Saunders, 1995:4333–4352.

History

▶ Right knee pain

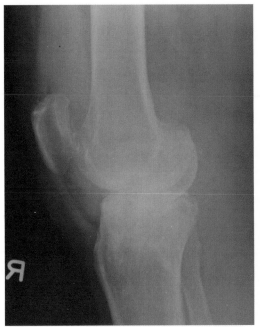

Figure 24.1

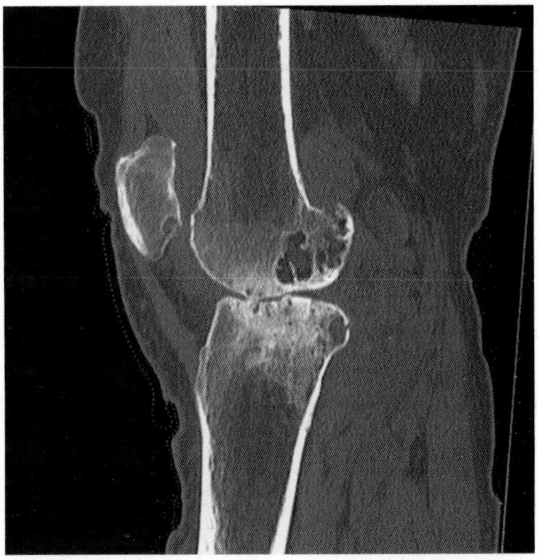

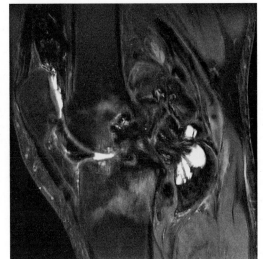

Figure 24.2

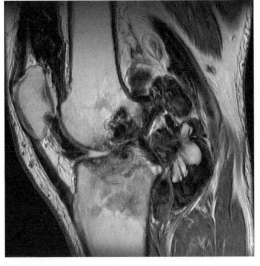

Figure 24.3

Figure 24.4

Case 24 Pigmented villonodular synovitis (PVNS), diffuse type

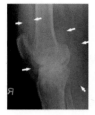 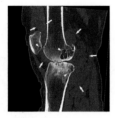 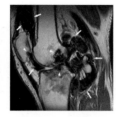 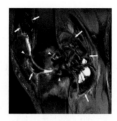

Figure 24.5　　　**Figure 24.6**　　　**Figure 24.7**　　　**Figure 24.8**

Findings

Figure 24.5 (lateral knee radiograph) shows abnormal soft tissue density within Hoffa's fat pad, the suprapatellar bursa and posterior joint (*white arrows*). Figure 24.6 (Sagittal CT) demonstrates lobulated soft tissue density extending within the suprapatellar bursa, Hoffa's fat pad, and posterior knee joint (*white arrows*) with subchondral lucencies/erosions with thin sclerotic margins (*arrowheads*) involving the posterior patella and the posterior femur and tibia. Figures 24.7 and 24.8 (Sagittal PD and PD FS MR images) depict persistent low-signal-intensity lobulated soft tissue material (*white arrows*) within the knee joint eroding subchondral regions of the patella, femur, and tibia (*arrowheads*).

Differential Diagnosis

The appearance is usually pathognomonic on MR; however, the following could be considered: nodular synovitis; osteochondromatosis; rheumatoid arthritis; hemangioma; amyloid (subchondral lesions on both sides of the joint).

Teaching Points

▶ PVNS is a vascular benign neoplastic proliferative disorder of the synovium of a joint (diffuse or local), extra-articular within a bursa (PVNB), or tendon sheath (PVNTS or giant cell tumor of the tendon sheath).

▶ Diffuse intra-articular PVNS is typically monoarticular, involving large joints (knee > hip). The masslike nature of PVNS results in subchondral lesions (chronic erosions) on both sides of the joint that mimic cysts. The CT appearance may also mimic an intraosseous mass, amyloidosis, chronic infection, or severe osteoarthritis on radiographs or CT however MRI helps to distinguish.

▶ PVNS tends to bleed, resulting in deposition of hemosiderin which is the cause for the pathognomonic decreased signal on both T1- and T2-weighted MR images and blooming artifact on GRE sequences in PVNS. Multinucleated cells with intra- and extracellular hemosiderin are noted on pathology.

▶ Lesions show peripheral or homogeneous contrast enhancement. Bone scan shows increased activity within the lesions on blood pool and flow due to increased vascularity.

▶ Rheumatoid arthritis (usually symmetric rather than monoarticular) and amyloid (subchondral lesions with soft tissue masses involving large joints) do not show low signal intensity on all MR sequences.

Management

MRI is critical in determining lesion extent. Treatment of choice is surgical excision, with other options including radiation therapy (external beam or radioisotope injection), pharmaceutical modulation of the disease, or a combination of the above in order to avoid recurrence. Recurrence rates are higher for diffuse intra-articular disease than localized types. Malignant transformation of PVNS is rare (3%); it can occur *de novo* or be associated with recurrent multiple episodic disease.

Further Readings

Jelinek J, Kransdorf M, Utz J, Berrey B, Thomson J, Heeken R, Radowich M. Imaging of pigmented villonodular synovitis with emphasis on MR imaging. *AJR Am J Roentgenol* 1989;*152*:337–342.

Murphey MD, Rhee JH, Lewis RB, Fanburg-Smith JC, Flemming DJ, Walker EA. From the Archives of the AFIP; Continuing Medical Education: Pigmented villonodular synovitis: Radiologic–pathologic correlation. *Radiographics* 2008;*28*(5):1493–1518.

History

▶ 35-year-old man with 3-year history of progressive left shoulder pain, swelling, and decreased range of motion

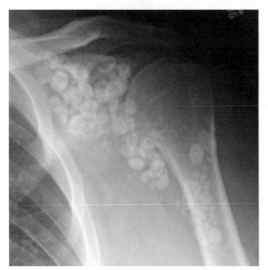

Figure 25.1

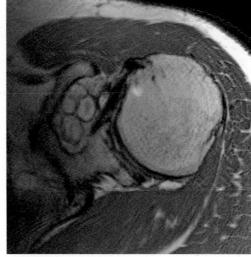

Figure 25.2

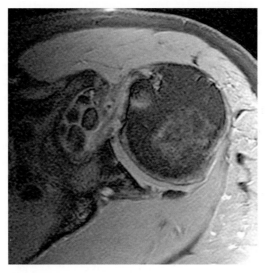

Figure 25.3

Case 25 Synovial osteochondromatosis (primary)

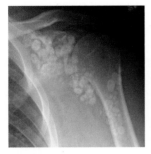
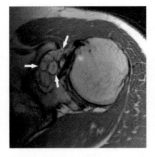
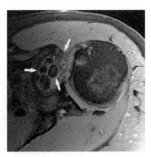

Figure 25.4   **Figure 25.5**   **Figure 25.6**

Findings

Figure 25.4 shows that multiple intra-articular osteochondral bodies are present within the left shoulder joint involving the subscapular recess, subcoracoid recess, and axillary pouch. Figure 25.5 (axial PD) confirms multiple high-signal-intensity (similar to intramedullary fat) rounded bodies with peripheral rims of thin low signal intensity (*white arrows*) within the subscapular recess. Figure 25.6 (AX FSPGR T1-weighted Fat Saturated post-gadolinium MR image) demonstrates fat saturation of multiple bodies (*white arrows*) within joint fluid/synovial thickening. No fracture or marked joint space narrowing is noted.

Differential Diagnosis

Secondary osteochondromatosis (post trauma or osteoarthritis); rheumatoid arthritis (Rice bodies); chondrosarcoma (rarely)

Teaching Points

▶ Synovial osteochondromatosis is an uncommon metaplastic synovial process resulting in nodular cartilage formation within the subsynovial soft tissues of a joint, bursa, or tendon sheath. It occurs most commonly within the hip, knee, elbow, and shoulder and is more frequent in men (2:1).

▶ There are primary and secondary types. Primary osteochondromatosis (no precipitating factors) has three phases: (1) Initial: Active intrasynovial disease without loose body formation; (2) Transition: Active intrasynovial proliferation and loose bodies with or without ossification; (3) Final: Multiple osteochondral loose bodies without intrasynovial proliferation. Secondary osteochondromatosis occurs more commonly and can be confirmed by associated findings of osteoarthritis, fracture, and/or articular surface degeneration.

▶ Intra-articular bodies may be entirely cartilaginous (seen as nodules and septations, which help distinguish it from a simple effusion), have central calcifications (confirmed by signal void on GRE MR images or "rings and arcs" on radiographs), or present as well-defined osteochondral bodies when advanced, as in this case.

▶ One third of cases never calcify; therefore, MRI is critical in diagnosis. CT is useful in confirming early calcification as well as extrinsic erosions, which can be seen in 20% to 30% of cases.

Management

In early stages, MRI is crucial for diagnosis. Radiographs better depict calcification. Treatment of primary type 1 and 2 is complete synovectomy; however, recurrence can occur in 3% to 23%. Radiographic follow-up is useful for identifying early recurrence. Phase 3 is treated with removal of intra-articular bodies without synovectomy.

Further Readings

Kransdorf MJ, Meis JM. From the Archives of the AFIP: Extraskeletal osseous and cartilaginous tumors of the extremities. *Radiographics* 1993;*13*:853–884.

Murphey MD, Vidal J, Fanburg-Smith J, Gajewski D. From the Archives of the AFIP: Imaging of synovial chondromatosis with radiologic–pathologic correlation. *Radiographics* 2007;*27*:1465–1488.

History

▶ Hand pain in two different patients

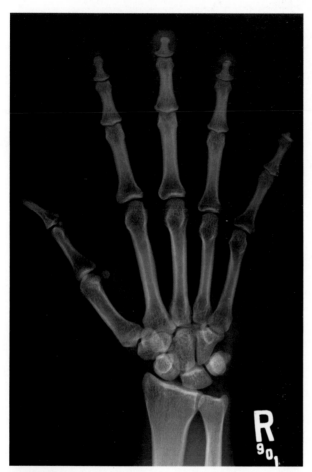

Figure 26.1

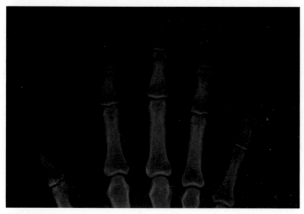

Figure 26.2

Case 26 Scleroderma

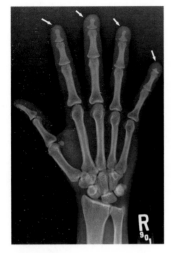

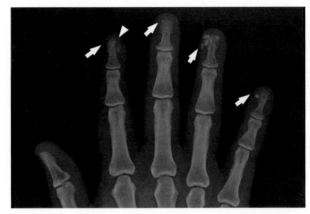

Figure 26.3   **Figure 26.4**

Findings

In the first patient (Fig. 26.3), marked erosion and resorption of the distal phalangeal tufts are noted with associated resorption of the soft tissues of the fingertips worse at the fifth digit (*small white arrows*).. In the second patient (Fig. 26.4), amorphous calcification in the soft tissues of the second through fifth fingertips with mild distal soft tissue resorption is noted (white arrows). Note also the erosive destruction of the second distal phalanx (*arrowhead*).

Differential Diagnosis

Mixed connective tissue disease; acro-osteolysis from drugs or frostbite

Teaching Points

▶ Scleroderma, or progressing systemic sclerosis, is a chronic disease that affects the skin, heart, lungs, gastrointestinal tract, kidneys, and musculoskeletal system.
▶ 46% of patients with this disease have arthropathy, which is limited to the hands and wrists.
▶ Resorption of the soft tissues of the fingertip with or without amorphous calcifications is the first visible radiographic change.
▶ Radiographic changes include:
  1. Resorption of the soft tissues of the fingertip
  2. Subcutaneous calcifications
  3. Erosions of the distal tufts (which may progress to resorb entire tuft)
  4. Acrosclerosis
▶ Occasional erosive disease of the IP joint or first CMC joints may be seen.

Management

Symptomatic treatment of arthropathy with focused treatment of other systemic symptoms. CREST syndrome includes scleroderma with calcinosis, Raynaud's phenomenon, esophageal dysfunction, sclerodactyly, and telangiectasias. The differential diagnosis includes systemic lupus erythematosus, polymyositis, and rheumatoid arthritis.

Further Readings

Brower AC, Flemming DJ. Collagen vascular diseases. In *Arthritis in Black and White*, 2nd ed. Philadelphia: Saunders, 1997:386–388.

Part II   **Lesions: Bone and Soft Tissue**

History

▶ 27-year-old man with left knee pain

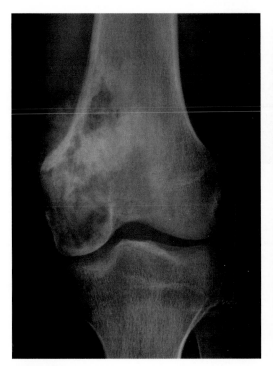

Figure 27.1

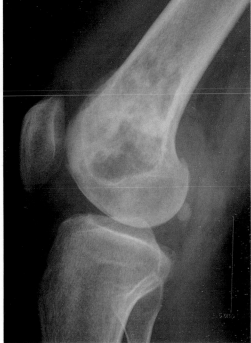

Figure 27.2

Case 27 Osteosarcoma

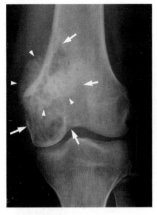

Figure 27.3

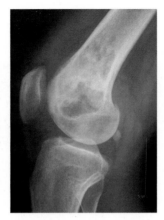

Figure 27.4

Findings

Radiographs of the left knee shown in Fig. 27.3 (AP) and 27.4 (lateral) reveal a large lytic lesion involving the medial femoral condyle and distal shaft (*arrows*) with a wide zone of transition and extension into the adjacent soft tissues. The lesion contains extensive, cloud-like densities compatible with osteoid matrix (*arrowheads*).

Differential Diagnosis

None

Teaching Points

▶ Osteosarcoma is the most common primary sarcoma of bone, with a peak incidence in the second decade. The most common sites of involvement include the distal femur, proximal tibia, and proximal humerus.

▶ These tumors are typically classified as intramedullary or surface lesions.

▶ Intramedullary types
  – Conventional (80% of all osteosarcomas)
  – Telangiectatic (may resemble an aneurysmal bone cyst)
  – Low grade
  – Small cell

▶ Surface types
  – Parosteal
  – Periosteal
  – High grade

▶ Typical radiographic findings include a poorly marginated, mixed lytic and sclerotic lesion (as in this case) with the areas of cloud-like sclerosis corresponding to osteoid matrix.

▶ Cortical breakthrough and extraosseous extension are common and are better assessed with MR imaging, the imaging modality of choice for local staging.

Management

Chemotherapy—often preoperative ("induction") and postoperative ("adjuvant")—combined with limb-salvage surgery, if possible. Amputation if unable to perform limb salvage.

Further Readings

Messerschmitt PJ, Garcia RM, Abdul-Karim FW, Greenfield EM, Getty PJ. Osteosarcoma. *J Am Acad Orthop Surg* 2009;*17*:515–527.

History

▸ 19-year-old male with dull localized pain involving the lower cervical spine

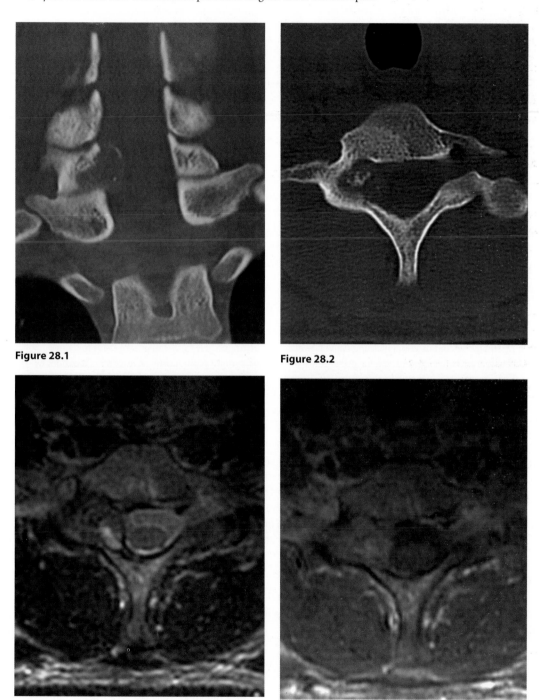

Figure 28.1

Figure 28.2

Figure 28.3

Figure 28.4

Case 28 Osteoblastoma of the right C7 pedicle

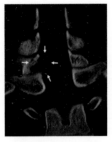 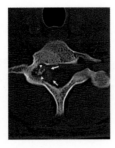 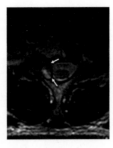 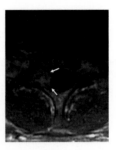

Figure 28.5   **Figure 28.6**   **Figure 28.7**   **Figure 28.8**

Findings

Figure 28.5 (coronal CT) shows a 2.0-cm expansile lesion of the right medial C7 pedicle with a thin sclerotic border and extension into the spinal canal (*white arrows*). Figure 28.6 (axial CT) better demonstrates the mass (*white arrows*) with central mineralization including a small central sequestrum (*arrowheads*), and left effacement of the cord and spinal canal. Axial T2-weighted and T1-weighted FS post-gadolinium MR images (Figs. 28.7 and 28.8) better depict the margins of the expansile lesion with mixed signal intensity (*white arrows*) and cord effacement.

Differential Diagnosis

Osteoid osteoma; foreign body reaction; Brodie's abscess; ABC or GCT; Brown tumor; fibrous dysplasia

Teaching Points

▶ Osteoblastoma is an uncommon slow-growing benign osseous lesion of young patients (80% <30 years of age).
▶ It resembles osteoid osteoma histologically; however, it is distinguished by its larger size (>1.5 to 2 cm) and characteristic symptoms of a localized dull ache, unlike the night pain of osteoid osteoma. Occasionally neurologic symptoms bring the patient to presentation secondary to neurovascular effacement or compression.
▶ Location: Approximately 40% occur in the spine (cervical > thoracic > lumbar), with a predilection for the posterior elements. Some cases extend to involve the vertebral body. 17% of spinal osteoblastomas occur in the sacrum. Femur and tibia (long tubular bones) are other sites (diaphysis>metaphysis).
▶ Imaging: Expansile geographic lucent intraosseous lesion with well-defined thin sclerotic margins and variable mineralization that may be confused with the ground-glass appearance of fibrous dysplasia or mixed arcs and rings of a chondroma. CT may be useful for delineating the cortical margin and mineralization as well as a rare but potential sequestrum similar to osteoid osteomas, as in this case. MR may also be useful for evaluating the size and extent of the lesion, particularly in patients presenting with neurologic symptoms An aneurysmal bone cyst (ABC) component may be seen in 10% to 15% of cases.
▶ Osteoblastomas demonstrate marked radionuclide uptake on bone scan. Large aggressive osteoblastomas can occur and are more difficult to treat.

Management

Excision is typically curative. Radiation may be included if the lesion is difficult to excise. Complex therapies are involved when the vertebral artery or nerve is involved and for aggressive osteoblastomas, as they may recur and have the potential for malignant transformation.

Further Readings

Jennin F, Bousson V, Parlier C, Jomaah N, Khanine V, Laredo JD. Bony sequestrum: a radiologic review. *Skeletal Radiol* 2011;*40*(8):963–975. Epub 2010 Jun 23.
Murphey MC, Andrews CL, Flemming DJ, Temple HT, Smith WS, Smirniotopoulos JG. From the archives of the AFIP. Primary tumors of the spine: Radiologic pathologic correlation. *Radiographics* 1996;38:835–844.

History

▶ Left shoulder pain

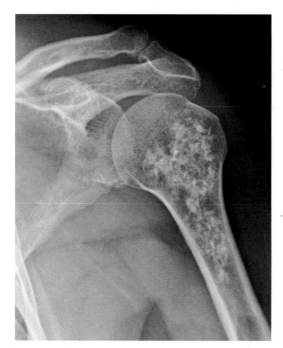

Figure 29.1

Case 29 Benign enchondroma

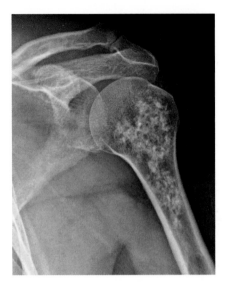

Figure 29.2

Findings

Flocculent, chondroid-appearing calcifications ("arcs and rings") within the proximal humerus. There is no evidence of endosteal scalloping or cortical breakthrough.

Differential Diagnosis

Low-grade chondrosarcoma; medullary infarction

Teaching Points

▶ Chondroid calcifications typically display an "arcs and rings" appearance.
▶ It can be impossible to distinguish a benign enchondroma from a low-grade chondrosarcoma radiographically, or even pathologically.
▶ Worrisome features include the following:
  1. Pain (often of months to years duration)
  2. Deep endosteal scalloping (greater than two thirds of cortical thickness)
  3. Cortical destruction and/or periosteal reaction
  4. Marked radionuclide uptake at scintigraphy (greater than the anterior iliac crest)
▶ A medullary infarction may display similar calcifications. Differentiation is most easily accomplished using MR imaging.

Management

Management of a benign-appearing chondroid lesion is controversial. Radiographic follow-up is often considered sufficient in the absence of pain. Some recommend complete curettage of any lesion over 7 cm with radiographic follow-up for up to two decades.

Further Readings

Brien EW, Mirra JM, Kerr. Benign and malignant cartilage tumors of bone and joint: their anatomic and theoretical basis with an emphasis on radiology, pathology and clinical biology—the intramedullary cartilage tumors. *Skeletal Radiol* 1997;26:325–353.
Murphey MD, Flemming DJ, Boyea SR, et. al. Enchondroma versus chondrosarcoma in the appendicular skeleton: differentiating features. *Radiographics* 1998;18:1213–1237.

History

▶ Chronic hand pain and deformity

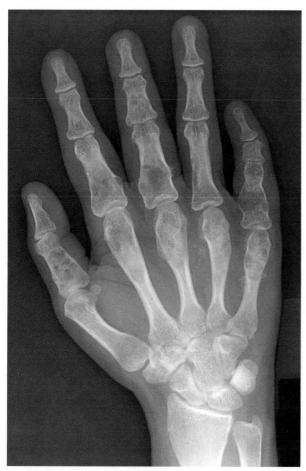

Figure 30.1

Case 30 Maffucci syndrome (multiple enchondromas and soft tissue hemangiomas)

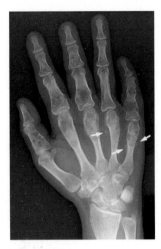

Figure 30.2

Findings

Figure 30.2 (AP radiograph of the right hand) demonstrates multiple, expansile lytic lesions within the metacarpals and phalanges as well as clusters of small phleboliths related to soft tissue hemangiomas (*arrows*).

Differential Diagnosis

None

Teaching Points

► Enchondromas are benign cartilaginous tumors that are commonly found within the tubular bones of the extremities. Typical radiographic findings include well-defined, often expansile, lytic lesions located centrally within the metaphysis or diaphysis of a long bone. They may result in prominent deformities.

► These lesions may be solitary or multiple (enchondromatosis).

► Ollier's disease refers to multiple enchondromas, often affecting predominantly one side of the body, whereas Maffucci syndrome is characterized by the combination of multiple enchondromas and soft tissue hemangiomas.

► Malignant transformation to a chondrosarcoma is rare in the case of a solitary enchondroma but is reported to occur in up to 30% to 50% of patients with Ollier's disease, and the incidence is higher in patients with Maffucci syndrome.

► While enchondromas are very common in the hands and feet, malignant transformation is extremely rare in these locations, even in the enchondromatosis syndromes.

Management

Usually just observational, though surgical resection may be necessary in cases of cosmetic deformity or malignant transformation.

Further Readings

Goto T, Motoi T, Komiya, et al. Chondrosarcoma of the hand secondary to multiple enchondromatosis; report of two cases. *Arch Orthop Trauma Surg.* 2003:*123*:42–47.

Pansuriya TC, Kroon HM, Bovee JVMG. Enchondromatosis: insights on the different subtypes. *Int J Clin Exp Pathol.* 2010;3:557–569.

History

▸ None provided

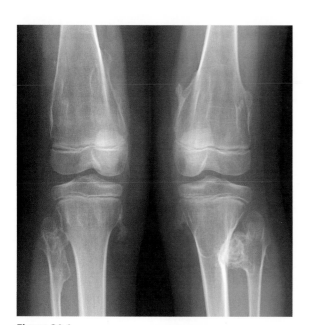

Figure 31.1

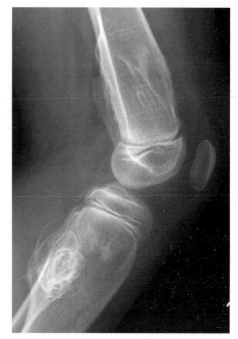

Figure 31.2

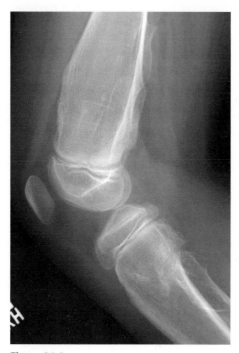

Figure 31.3

Case 31 Multiple hereditary exostoses

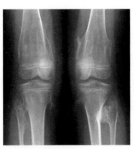
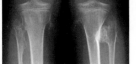
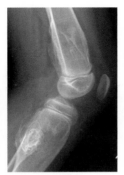

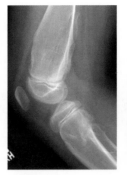
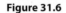
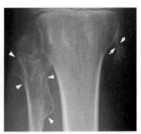

Figure 31.4   **Figure 31.5**   **Figure 31.6**   **Figure 31.7**

Findings

Figures 31.4 (PA), and 31.5 and 31.6 (lateral views of both knees) reveal multiple osseous excrescences involving the bones of both knees. Figure 31.7 (coned-down view of the proximal tibia and fibula) demonstrates the thin stalk (arrows) of a pedunculated osteochondroma as well as the broad involvement and cortical contiguity of the sessile fibular lesions, *arrowheads*).

Differential Diagnosis

Solitary lesion: prior, healed avulsion fracture; "tug" lesion related to chronic avulsive changes at a tendon insertion. Multiple lesions: none.

Teaching Points

▶ Osteochondromas (exostoses) are cartilaginous tumors of bone that may be solitary or multiple, as in this case (multiple hereditary exostoses).

▶ Two types are seen. A pedunculated lesion arises from the bone via a relatively narrow stalk, whereas a sessile type demonstrates a broader attachment.

▶ These can arise from any bone, and when involving a long bone, they most commonly arise from the metaphysis and are pointed away from the adjacent joint.

▶ Important findings to look for on imaging studies include a smooth, contiguous transition from the normal cortex to that of the lesion and contiguity between the marrow cavities of the bone and lesion.

▶ Complications of these lesions that may produce pain include the following:
  ▪ Impingement of adjacent bones or soft tissues
  ▪ Fracture (especially the pedunculated type)
  ▪ Development of overlying bursitis
  ▪ Malignant transformation (rare)

Management

Clinical and radiographic monitoring; surgical therapy for painful lesions

Further Readings

Lee KCY, Davies AM, Cassar-Pullicino VN. Imaging the complications of osteochondromas. *Clin Radiol* 2002;*57*:18–28.

Ozaki T, Kawai A, Sugihara S, Takei Y, Inone H. Multiple osteocartilaginous exostosis: a follow-up study. *Arch Orthop Trauma Trauma Surg* 1996;*115*:255–261.

History

▶ Young patient with right hip pain

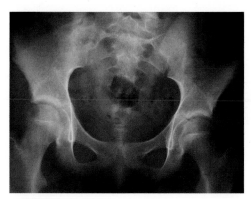

Figure 32.1

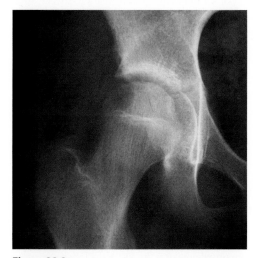

Figure 32.2

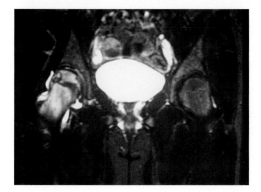

Figure 32.3

Case 32 Chondroblastoma, right femoral head

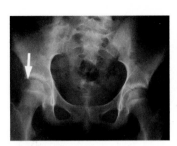

Figure 32.4

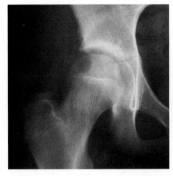

Figure 32.5

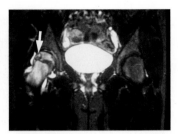

Figure 32.6

Findings

Figures 32.4 (AP image of the pelvis) and 32.5 (coned-down view of the right hip) demonstrate a relatively well-circumscribed, rounded lytic lesion in the lateral aspect of the capital femoral epiphysis (*arrow*). Figure 32.6 (coronal STIR [inversion recovery] image of the pelvis) confirms the presence of the lesion in the femoral epiphysis (*arrow*) and also reveals extensive marrow edema throughout the femoral head and neck as well as a moderate-sized joint effusion.

Differential Diagnosis

Brodie's abscess

Teaching Points

▶ Chondroblastoma is a benign cartilaginous tumor that arises in secondary ossification centers (epiphyses and apophyses), most frequently in the proximal and distal portions of the femur, the proximal tibia, and the proximal humerus.
▶ Although this lesion is usually seen in skeletally immature patients, it may also be found after physeal closure.
▶ The typical radiographic appearance of a chondroblastoma is that of a relatively well-defined lytic lesion within an epiphysis or apophysis.
▶ Radionuclide bone scan will demonstrate a focus of intense abnormal uptake at the site of the lesion.
▶ MR imaging may be misleading since this lesion is usually associated with extensive edema-like signal abnormality with the adjacent marrow, as in this case, mimicking a more aggressive lesion. Similar findings are seen in other benign lesions such as osteoid osteoma and Langerhans cell histiocytosis.

Management

Complete surgical curettage of the lesion

Further Readings

James SL, Panicek DM, Davies AM. Bone marrow oedema associated with benign and malignant bone tumors. *Eur J Radiol.* 2008;67:11–21.

History

▶ 44-year-old man with left shoulder mass and pain

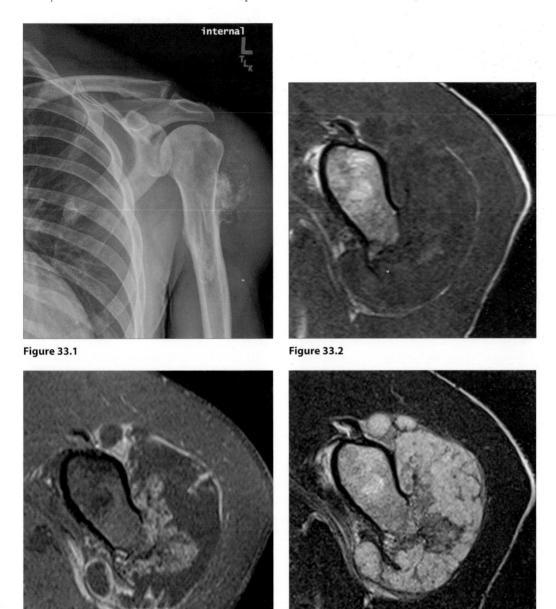

Figure 33.1

Figure 33.2

Figure 33.3

Figure 33.4

Case 33 Secondary chondrosarcoma (multiple hereditary exostoses with malignant transformation of osteochondroma)

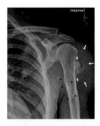 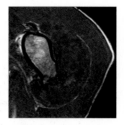 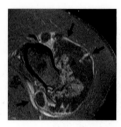 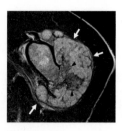

Figure 33.5   **Figure 33.6**   **Figure 33.7**   **Figure 33.8**

Findings

Figure 33.5 shows lobular ring and arc mineralization (*white arrows*) surrounding the supralateral left humeral metadiaphysis at the level of a focal contiguous intramedullary excrescence of bone (osteochondroma) (*small white arrows*). Two other osteochondromas are present within the medial humeral metadiaphysis and anterior left third rib (*black arrowheads*). Figure 33.6 (axial T1-weighted MR image) demonstrates a soft tissue mass of intermediate signal intensity with mild heterogeneity surrounding the proximal humeral diametaphysis laterally with loss of the normal cortex at the neck of the underlying osteochondroma (*arrowheads*). Figure 33.7 (axial T1-weighted FS post-gadolinium) and 33.8 (axial T2-weighted images) demonstrate diffuse high-signal (T2)-intensity lobulated mass (*white arrows*) with only peripheral lobular and septal enhancement of the soft tissue component post contrast administration (*black arrows*) with central lower myxoid signal material and lobular enhancement of the irregular area of mineralization at the region of the cartilage cap (*black arrowheads*).

Differential Diagnosis

Osteochondroma; osteosarcoma; infection; tumoral calcinosis; chondroma

Teaching Points

▶ Osteochondromas may be solitary or multiple, the latter being associated with hereditary multiple exostoses (HME), an autosomal dominant syndrome. Complications associated with osteochondromas include deformity (cosmetic and osseous), fracture, vascular compromise, neurologic sequelae, overlying bursa formation, and malignant transformation. Complications are more frequent in patients with HME.

▶ Malignant transformation occurs in1% of patients with solitary osteochondromas and in 3% to 5% of patients with HME. Malignancy usually occurs within the overlying cartilage cap. Continued lesion growth and a hyaline cartilage cap thicker than 1.5 cm, after skeletal maturity, suggest malignant transformation.

▶ Secondary chondrosarcoma (as in this case) represents 8% of all chondrosarcomas.

▶ Features associated with malignant transformation include irregular prominent arc and ring mineralization extending from the region of the osteochondroma cap with associated soft tissue mass and pain. The peripheral lobular enhancement of the soft tissue component is typical of chondroid malignancies with high T2 signal and low CT attenuation due to high water content, with associated scattered mineralization and erosion or destruction of adjacent bone.

Management

Secondary chondrosarcoma, particularly in HME, requires MR and CT imaging for further evaluation and radiographs or bone scan to assess for other osteochondromas. Metastatic disease is rare. Typical location is lung, requiring chest radiograph and CT for evaluation. Wide surgical resection and limb salvage without radiation or chemotherapy is the preferred treatment. Prognosis is good, with 70% to 90% long-term survival, with the exception of dedifferentiated types, which have a worse prognosis.

Further Readings

Brien EW, Mirra JM, Kerr. Benign and malignant cartilage tumors of bone and joint: their anatomic and theoretical basis with an emphasis on radiology, pathology and clinical biology—the intramedullary cartilage tumors. *Skeletal Radiol* 1997;26:325–353.

Murphey MD, Choi JJ, Kransdorf MJ, et al. Imaging of osteochondroma: variants and complications with radiologic–pathologic correlation. *Radiographics* 2000;20(5):1407–1434.

History

▶ 58-year-old woman with left knee pain

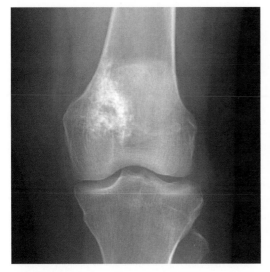

Figure 34.1

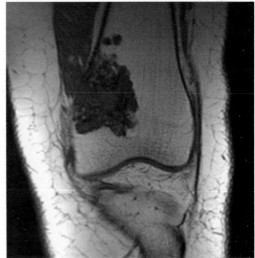

Figure 34.2

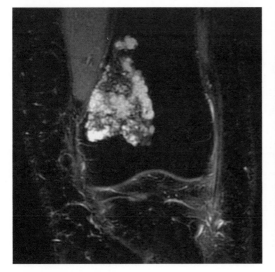

Figure 34.3

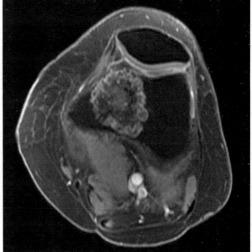

Figure 34.4

Case 34 Low-grade chondrosarcoma

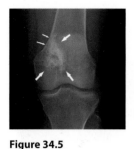
Figure 34.5

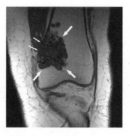
Figure 34.6

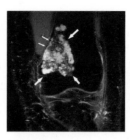
Figure 34.7

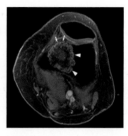
Figure 34.8

Findings

Figure 34.5 (AP radiograph) shows ring and arc lobular mineralization within the distal left femoral diametaphysis (*white arrows*) with endosteal scalloping of the medial femoral cortex (*small arrows*). Figures 34.6 (coronal T1) and 34.7 (Coronal STIR) MR images demonstrate a 5.9 × 3.3-cm lobulated intramedullary metadiaphyseal femoral mass (*white arrows*), predominantly T1 hypointense and STIR heterogeneously hyperintense, demonstrating both T1 and STIR ring and arc-like marked hypointensities consistent with mineralization. MR confirms endosteal scalloping (*small arrows*), extension into the epiphysis abutting the intercondylar notch without soft tissue extension, periosteal reaction, surrounding bone marrow edema, or fracture. Figure 34.8 (axial FSPGR post-gadolinium image) shows ring-like enhancement of the peripheral lobules (*arrowheads*) and marked thinning of the anterior/medial cortex of the distal femur (*arrows*).

Differential Diagnosis

Enchondroma; medullary infarction

Teaching Points

► Chondroid calcifications typically display an "arc and ring" appearance.
► It can be impossible to distinguish a benign enchondroma from a low-grade chondrosarcoma radiographically, or even pathologically.
► Worrisome features include:
  1. Pain (often of months to years duration)
  2. Deep endosteal scalloping (greater than two thirds of cortical thickness)
  3. Cortical destruction and/or periosteal reaction
  4. Marked radionuclide uptake at scintigraphy (greater than the anterior iliac crest)
► A medullary infarction may display similar apparent mineralization on radiographs. Differentiation is most easily accomplished using MR imaging.

Management

A chondroid-appearing lesion with associated clinical pain and suggestion of endosteal scalloping and large size on radiographs requires MR or CT imaging for further evaluation. Tissue biopsy is recommended to confirm or exclude true malignancy. Chondrosarcoma typically requires complete resection and close imaging follow-up to exclude recurrence. Low grade cartilage lesions may be monitored at close intervals.

Further Readings

Brien EW, Mirra JM, Kerr. Benign and malignant cartilage tumors of bone and joint: their anatomic and theoretical basis with an emphasis on radiology, pathology and clinical biology—the intramedullary cartilage tumors. *Skeletal Radiol* 1997;*26*:325–353.
Murphey MD, Flemming DJ, Boyea SR, et. al. Enchondroma versus chondrosarcoma in the appendicular skeleton: differentiating features. *Radiographics* 1998;*18*:1213–1237.
Murphey MD, Walker EA, Wilson AJ, et al. From the archives of the AFIP: imaging of primary chondrosarcoma: radiologic–pathologic correlation. *Radiographics* 2003;*23*(5):1245–1278.

History

▶ 62-year-old man with history of prior right thigh mass, now with increased fullness in the proximal right thigh

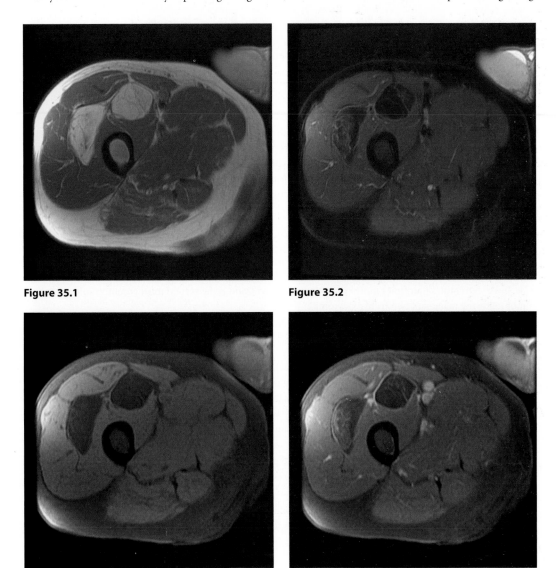

Figure 35.1

Figure 35.2

Figure 35.3

Figure 35.4

Case 35 Well-differentiated low-grade liposarcoma (recurrent)

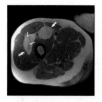 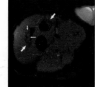 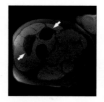 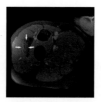

Figure 35.5   **Figure 35.6**   **Figure 35.7**   **Figure 35.8**

Findings

MR images of the right thigh (Fig. 35.5, axial, T1-weighted; Fig. 35.6, STIR; Fig. 35.7; and Fig. 35.8, FSPGR Fat Saturated pre and post gadolinium administration respectively) demonstrate a bilobed, predominantly fatty mass within the deep musculature of the proximal thigh, predominantly high signal intensity on T1 and low signal intensity on STIR (*white arrows*). Internal lateral heterogeneous focal and septal areas of lower T1 intensity and corresponding high STIR signal intensity (*small white arrows*) demonstrate enhancement post gadolinium administration. No calcification was noted on CT (not shown).

Differential Diagnosis

Fatty replacement of muscle; lipoma

Teaching Points

▶ Liposarcoma accounts for 16% to 18% of all soft tissue sarcomas, tends to occur in the extremities (65% to 77%; lower extremities four times more common than upper), and is the second most common soft tissue tumor following malignant fibrous histiocytoma.

▶ It can be differentiated from simple lipoma by the following imaging characteristics:
  1. Lack of homogeneous fatty tissue
  2. Thickened septations
  3. Presence of nonadipose soft tissue nodules
  4. Enhancement of soft tissue components, confirming nonadipose tissue
  5. Large size (greater than 10 cm is suspicious for liposarcoma and should be followed)

▶ Liposarcomas occur in older patient and are typically painless. Pain/tenderness occurs in 10% to 15%.

▶ Classification of liposarcomas (four categories according to WHO):
  ■ *Well differentiated* (most common type, and what is shown in this case): Low-grade sarcoma that recurs locally but does not metastasize and is considered atypical if superficial in location. Majority are >75% fat. May have calcifications (10% to 15%). Good prognosis.
  ■ *Dedifferentiated*: Closely related to the well-differentiated type. A bimorphic lesion with high-grade pleomorphic sarcoma of nonadipose cells usually focal and juxtaposed with low-grade well-differentiated liposarcoma.
  ■ *Myxoid*: Intermediate grade may coexist with hypercellular high grade. Predilection for extrapulmonary metastases. Central areas of fatty differentiation (<25% of mass) best seen on MR. Currently includes round cell liposarcoma category.
  ■ *Pleomorphic*: High grade and least common type

Management

Advanced imaging (CT/MR) helps distinguish fat from nonadipose components, with contrast confirming soft tissue components and the extent of the lesion. Biopsy for tissue confirmation should be performed under CT/MR or US guidance to the areas of nonadipose tissue. CT of the chest and abdomen should be performed to evaluate for metastatic disease in subtypes other than well-differentiated liposarcoma.

Further Readings

Kransdorf MJ, Murphey MD. *Lipomatous tumors. In Imaging of Soft Tissue Tumors*, 2nd ed. Philadelphia: Lippincott Williams and Wilkins, 2006:125–149.

Murphey MD, Arcara LK, Fanburg-Smith J. Imaging of musculoskeletal liposarcoma with radiologic–pathologic correlation. *Radiographics* 2005;1371–1395.

History

▸ 10-year-old boy with 2 days of lower right quadrant abdominal pain

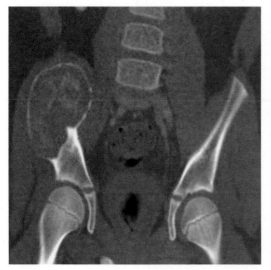

Figure 36.1

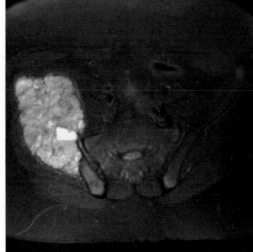

Figure 36.2

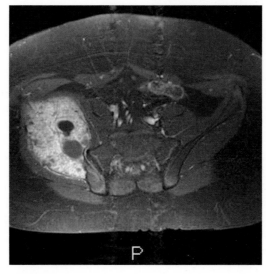

Figure 36.3

Case 36   Aneurysmal bone cyst (ABC)

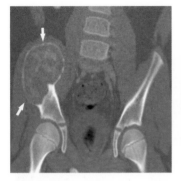
Figure 36.4

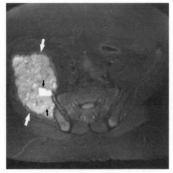
Figure 36.5

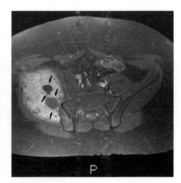
Figure 36.6

Findings

Figure 36.4 (coronal CT) depicts an expansile intraosseous predominantly lytic lesion of the right iliac bone (*white arrows*) with mild heterogeneous internal matrix. Figures 36.5 (axial T2 FS) and 36.6 (T1 FS post gadolinium) depict an expansile intraosseous lesion (*white arrows*) with fluid–fluid levels (blood-filled cystic cavities) (*black arrows*) with diffuse enhancement and septa throughout the majority of the lesion, with regions of nonenhancement. A thin cortical rim remains.

Differential Diagnosis

Giant cell tumor; telangiectatic osteosarcoma; Ewing sarcoma (location good but typically no fluid–fluid levels); giant osteoblastoma with secondary ABC or giant cell tumor; expansile metastasis; hemophilia (pseudotumor)

Teaching Points

▶ ABC is an expansile intraosseous benign bone lesion that is most common in the posterior elements of the spine (thoracic > lumbar > cervical > sacrum) but can occur in the long bones or pelvis.
▶ It is characterized by "fluid–fluid" levels on MR, CT, or US due to blood-filled cavities, expansion, and a thin remaining cortical rim.
▶ One third of cases have co existing lesions—giant cell tumor (most common), osteoblastoma, chondroblastoma, or telengiectatic osteosarcoma (all of which can have fluid–fluid levels).
▶ Age group: 5 to 20 years of age, with a slight female predilection
▶ Imaging: Expansile geographic lucent intraosseous cystic-appearing lesion with thin cortical rim, multiple fluid–fluid levels and septa on MR or CT accounting for heterogeneous enhancement pattern due to blood with potential for increased blood signal intensity areas on T1-weighted images. Intense radiotracer uptake on bone scan at the periphery of the lesion, known as the "doughnut sign," is seen in 64% of cases.

Management

Treatment includes presurgical selective arterial embolization, intralesional excision and curettage, bone grafting, and fusion if instability is evident.

Further Readings

Kransdorf MJ, Sweet DE. Aneurysmal bone cyst: concept, controversy, clinical presentation, and imaging. *AJR Am J Roentgenol* 1995;*164*(3):573–580.
Murphey MC, Andrews CL, Flemming DJ, Temple HT, Smith WS, Smirniotopoulos JG. From the archives of the AFIP. Primary tumors of the spine: Radiologic–pathologic correlation. *Radiographics* 1996;*38*:835–844.
Rodellac MH, Feydy A, Larousserie F, Anract P, Campagna R, Babinet A, Zins M, Drape JL. Diagnostic imaging of solitary tumors of the spine: What to do and say. *Radiographics* 2008;*28*:1091–1041.

History

▶ 25-year-old man with knee pain

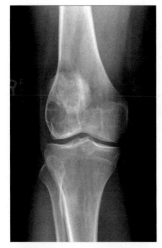

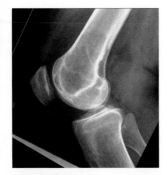

Figure 37.1

Figure 37.2

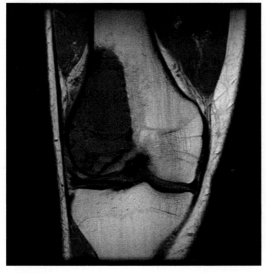

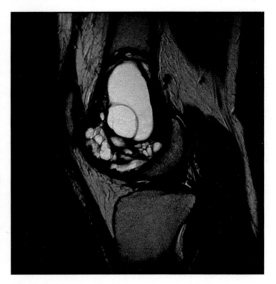

Figure 37.3

Figure 37.4

Case 37 Giant cell tumor of the distal femur

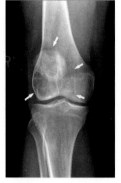

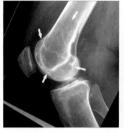

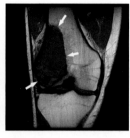

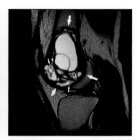

Figure 37.5　　　　**Figure 37.6**　　　　**Figure 37.7**　　　　**Figure 37.8**

Findings

Figures 37.5 and 37.6 (AP and lateral knee radiographs) demonstrate an eccentric bubbly lytic intramedullary lesion with small septations within the distal meta-epiphysis of the femur without definite cortical breakthrough or internal matrix on radiographs (*white arrows*). Figures 37.7 and 37.8 (coronal T1 and sagittal T2 fat-saturated MR images) demonstrate a lower-signal-intensity T1 heterogeneous septated intramedullary lesion with endosteal scalloping and mild cortical permeation without fracture. Fluid–fluid levels are present on the T2 fat-saturated sequences (*small white arrows*). No definite soft tissue component is noted and the lesion does not cross the joint.

Differential Diagnosis

Aneurysmal bone cyst (ABC); telangectatic osteosarcoma; chondroblastoma; fibroxanthoma (radiographs only); infection; hemophilia pseudotumor; large geode (radiographs only, in appropriate setting)

Teaching Points

▶ Eccentric bubbly lytic bone lesion with septations
▶ Well-defined with cortical permeation with or without fracture
▶ No sclerotic border (helps exclude fibroxanthoma and geode)
▶ Location: Metaphysis extending to epiphysis and subchondral bone
▶ MRI: fluid–fluid levels (also seen in ABC, chondroblastoma, and telangiectatic osteosarcoma)
▶ Solid components may demonstrate low to intermediate T2 signal intensity. Locally aggressive lesion that can have a soft tissue component – important to identify soft tissue component and extent of lesion (i.e., across a joint) as these findings may change management.
▶ May coexist with aneurysmal bone cyst or chondroblastoma
▶ Age group: Closed physes, age >20 years
▶ Malignant giant cell tumor accounts for 5% to 10% of all giant cell tumors and is usually secondary to previous irradiation of benign giant cell tumor.

Management

Biopsy must be directed at the solid components of the lesion, best demonstrated on CT or MRI, to obtain diagnostic tissue. Treatment of giant cell tumor usually consists of surgical resection and curettage. Recurrence is seen in 2% to 25% of cases

Further Readings

Murphey MD, Nomikos GC, Flemming DJ, Gannon FH, Temple HT, Kransdorf MJ. Imaging of giant cell tumor and giant cell reparative granuloma of bone: radiologic–pathologic correlation. *Radiographics* 2001;*21*:1283–1309.
Stacy G, Peabody T, Dixon L. Mimics on radiography of giant cell tumor of bone. *AJR Am J Roentgenol* 2003;*181*:1583–1589.

History

▶ 16-year-old with ankle pain s/p fall

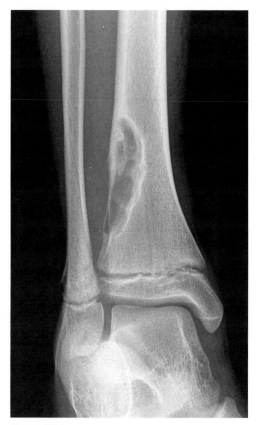

Figure 38.1

Case 38 Fibroxanthoma

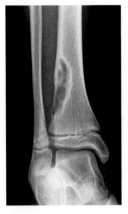
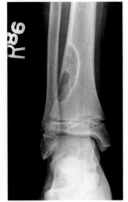

Figure 38.2   **Figure 38.3**

Findings

Figure 38.2 (ankle radiograph) shows an eccentrically located, cortically based intramedullary, lobulated lesion within the distal diametaphysis of the tibia that exhibits central lucency and a well-defined sclerotic border. No periosteal reaction, fracture, or soft tissue abnormality is seen. Figure 38.3 in another patient demonstrates increased central sclerosis within a similar lesion which is characteristic of a healing fibroxanthoma.

Differential Diagnosis

Appearance is usually characteristic, but the differential diagnosis may include chondromyxoid fibroma or fibrous dysplasia.

Teaching Points

► Fibroxanthoma is the preferred terminology for the benign fibrous lesion of bone: nonossifying fibroma (NOF) (>3 cm) and fibrous cortical defect (<3 cm).
► These lesions are typically solitary, eccentric, diametaphyseal, cortically based intramedullary lesions with central lucency and a well-demarcated sclerotic rim.
► They are typically asymptomatic and only noted incidentally for other imaging reasons.
► They may occasionally present with microfracture with secondary pain, swelling, and periosteal reaction. The lesions are at increased risk for fracture if they involve >50% of the width of the involved bone.
► Fibroxanthomas heal by sclerosis over time and may disappear by the mid-twenties.
► CT demonstrates similar appearance to radiographs. MR may be more sensitive for early microfracture. Typical MR appearance is of well-defined low-signal margin and with central mixed fat and fibrous signal without peripheral edema or soft tissue mass.
► Multiple fibroxanthomas can occur. There are rare reports of association with neurofibromatosis. The presence of extraskeletal congenital anomalies (café-au-lait spots, mental retardation, hypogonadism or cryptorchidism, ocular abnormality, cardiovascular malformations) in association with multiple nonossifying fibroxanthomas constitutes the clinical and radiologic spectrum known as Jaffe-Campanacci syndrome.

Management

Typically no treatment for asymptomatic lesions. If associated pain without trauma, evaluation of fracture and treatment of fracture as appropriate. If multiple lesions, one must assess for neurofibromatosis or Jaffe-Campanacci syndrome.

Further Readings

Kumar R, Madewell J, Lindell M, Swischuk L. Fibrous lesions of bones. *Radiographics* 1990;*10*:237–256.
Smith SE. Imaging in fibrous cortical defect and non-ossifying fibroma. *Emedicine Radiology* 2003;*4*(7).

History

▶ Right hip pain

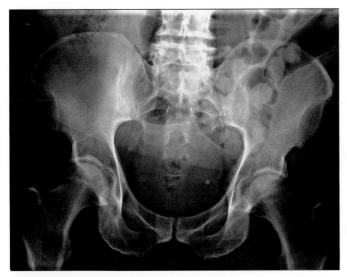

Figure 39.1

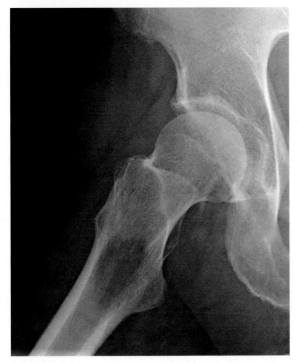

Figure 39.2

Case 39   Metastatic lung cancer, right femur

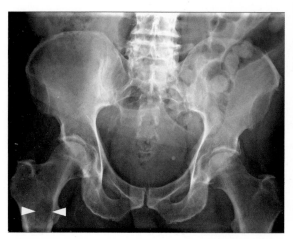

Figure 39.3

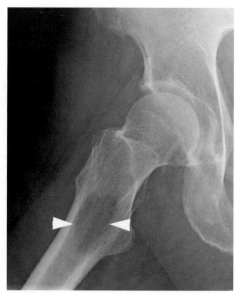

Figure 39.4

Findings

Figures 39.3 (AP pelvis) and 39.4 (frog-leg lateral view of the right hip) reveal an ill-defined lytic lesion in the proximal femur adjacent to the lesser trochanter (*arrowheads*).

Differential Diagnosis

Other aggressive lesions such as myeloma, lymphoma, or other primary bone neoplasm. Osteomyelitis could have a similar appearance.

Teaching Points

▶ The radiographic findings of a focal lytic lesion with ill-defined margins (wide zone of transition) suggest an "aggressive" bone lesion.
▶ In a patient over the age of 40, metastases and myeloma should top the list of differential possibilities, even in the case of a solitary lesion.
▶ A radionuclide bone scan provides a rapid survey of the entire skeleton and is useful for identifying additional lesions.
▶ MR imaging is the best modality for local staging, and in some centers whole body MRI is used rather than a bone scan, given its greater sensitivity for bone lesions.
▶ In a patient with a newly discovered primary neoplasm, the detection of an osseous metastasis is important for accurate staging, and image-guided biopsy often plays an important role in the initial workup of these patients.

Management

Demonstration of metastatic disease will dramatically alter the therapy for most tumors (toward medical therapy and away from surgical management).

Further Readings

Miller TT. Bone tumors and tumorlike conditions: analysis with conventional radiography. *Radiology* 2008;246:662–674.

History

▶ 68-year-old woman with knee pain and swelling

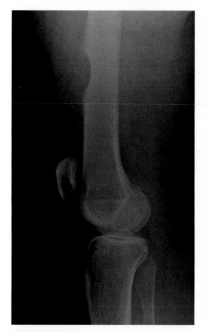

Figure 40.1

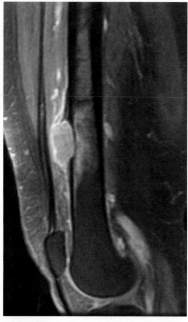

Figure 40.2

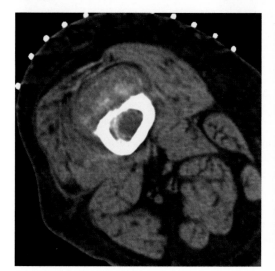

Figure 40.3

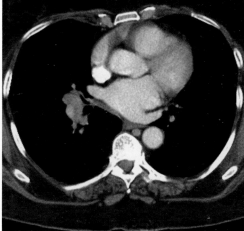

Figure 40.4

Case 40 Cortical metastasis (femur), secondary to primary bronchogenic carcinoma

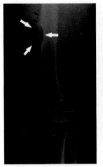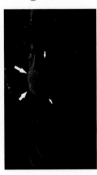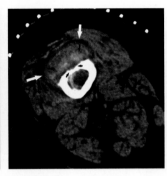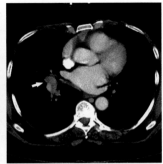

Figure 40.5   **Figure 40.6**   **Figure 40.7**   **Figure 40.8**

Findings

Figure 40.5 (lateral femur radiograph) shows a concave "cookie bite"-appearing anterior distal femoral diaphyseal cortical defect/destruction (*white arrows*) with associated periosteal reaction and apparent uplifting of the superior and inferior cortical bone (*small black arrows*). Figure 40.6 (post gadolinium FSPGR Fat Saturated sagittal MR) confirms a homogeneous oval smooth soft tissue lesion invading the anterior femoral cortex that demonstrates diffuse enhancement after the administration of intravenous contrast (*white arrows*). Associated bone marrow edema within the distal femoral diaphysis is present (*small white arrows*). Figure 40.7 (axial CT) best demonstrates anterior femoral cortical destruction with associated periosteal reaction (*black arrows*). Figure 40.8 (chest CT) shows a right parahilar irregular soft tissue mass (*white arrow*).

Differential Diagnosis

Fairly pathognomonic but could include: osteomyelitis; parosteal sarcoma (over time); periosteal sarcoma; foreign body granuloma

Teaching Points

▶ *Radiographs*: Concave cortical erosion within the *diaphysis* of a long bone with associated periosteal reaction and soft tissue mass has been described in association with bronchogenic carcinoma metastases and is termed the "cookie bite" sign. Other extraosseous primary tumors may have metastases to cortex (renal cell, breast, melanoma, epidermoid).

▶ *CT and MR*: Utilized to better delineate cortical lesion, to evaluate for intramedullary edema, to visualize the presence as well as extent of associated soft tissue mass, which is best seen on post-contrast imaging, and to plan for biopsy

▶ *Nuclear medicine*: Bone scan is useful to assess for other metastatic foci with diffuse increased uptake.

Management

Evaluation of the chest with radiographs and CT is paramount, as this usually is seen with primary bronchogenic carcinoma. Biopsy to confirm diagnosis. PET-CT may be of benefit to evaluate for other metastatic lesions.

Further Readings

Deutch A, Resnik D. Eccentric cortical metastases to the skeleton from bronchogenic carcinoma. *Radiology* 1980;*137*:49–52.
Hendrix RW, Rogers L, Davis T. Cortical bone metastases. *Radiology* 1991;*181*;409–413.
Snoeckx A, Vanhoenacker FM, Petre C, Parizel PM. Images in Clinical Radiology: Cookie bite lesion. *JBR-BTR* 2006;*89*:48.

History

▶ Low back and pelvic pain

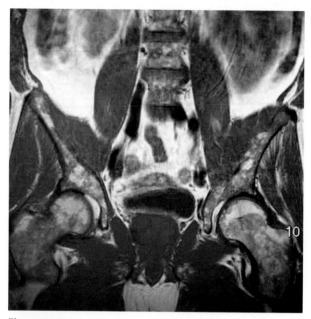

Figure 41.1

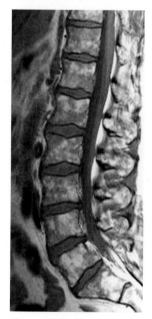

Figure 41.2

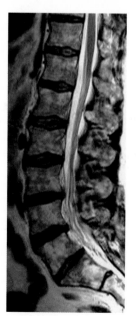

Figure 41.3

Case 41 Multiple myeloma (variegated pattern)

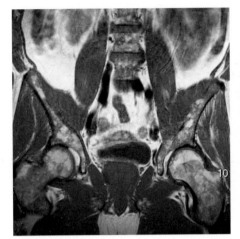

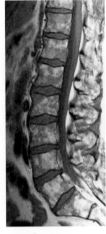

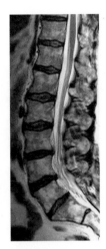

Figure 41.4

Figure 41.5

Figure 41.6

Findings

Figure 41.4 (coronal T1-weighted image) reveals patchy areas of intermediate to low signal intensity throughout the marrow of the lumbar spine, pelvis, and proximal portions of the femurs. Sagittal images of the lumbar spine in Figures 41.5 (T1-weighted) and 41.6 (T2-weighted) show similar, variegated areas of abnormal signal intensity throughout the marrow of the lower thoracic and lumbar spine.

Differential Diagnosis

Osseous metastases

Teaching Points

▶ Multiple myeloma is a neoplastic condition of the marrow (plasma cells) and is the most common primary malignant tumor of bone. It typically affects patients over the age of 40.

▶ The axial skeleton, pelvis, and proximal extremities are most commonly involved.

▶ Radiographic findings may include a single lytic lesion, numerous small "punched-out" lytic lesions, or diffuse osteoporosis.

▶ Whole-body CT has been advocated as a more sensitive alternative to the classic radiographic skeletal series.

▶ Radionuclide bone scanning is often normal, and although PET scanning is relatively insensitive for detecting diffuse involvement, it may be helpful in identifying focal lesions.

▶ Several patterns have been described on MR imaging:
  – A "normal" scan in which the tumor burden is so low that it can't be differentiated from normal hematopoietic ("red") marrow
  – Focal, geographic lesions
  – Patchy, "variegated" foci (as in this case)
  – Diffuse signal abnormality throughout the marrow (poorer prognosis)

▶ The imaging findings are often indistinguishable from osseous metastases, and an accurate diagnosis may require correlation with serum electrophoresis and/or biopsy.

Management

Chemotherapy and possibly autologous bone marrow transplantation

Further Readings

Delorme S, Baur-Melnyk A. Imaging in multiple myeloma. *Eur J Radiol* 2009;70:401–408.

History

▶ 77-year-old woman with pain, swelling, and decreased range of motion of the left shoulder

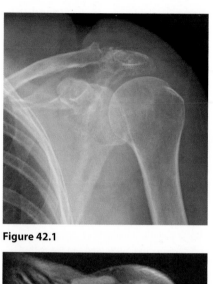

Figure 42.1

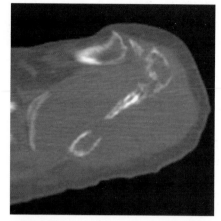

Figure 42.2

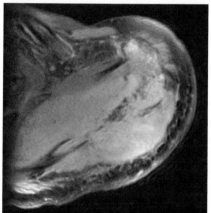

Figure 42.3

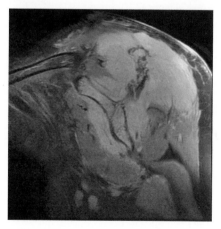

Figure 42.4

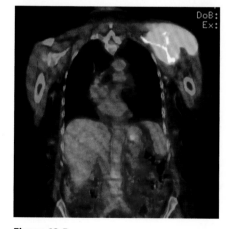

Figure 42.5

Case 42   Lymphoma (B-cell large-cell type, non-Hodgkin's) of the scapula

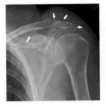
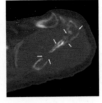
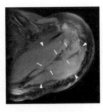
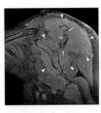
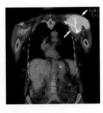

| **Figure 42.6** | **Figure 42.7** | **Figure 42.8** | **Figure 42.9** | **Figure 42.10** |

Findings

Figure 42.6 (AP radiograph of the left shoulder) shows moth-permeative destruction of the left acromion and superior scapula (*white arrows*) with associated periosteal reaction/sclerosis. Figure 42.7 (axial CT of the left shoulder) better demonstrates permeative destruction of the superior left scapula and acromion (*small arrows*) with extensive soft tissue component involving all rotator cuff muscles. Figures 42.8 and 42.9 (axial and sagittal proton density fat-saturated MR) better demonstrate the extensive infiltrative soft tissue mass (high signal intensity) involving the rotator cuff muscles (*arrowheads*). The high signal soft tissue (ST) component is contiguous with the destructive intramedullary scapular lesion via multiple vascular channels or defects within the cortex (*small arrows*).Figure 42.10 (fused FDG PET-CT) shows marked abnormal increased uptake within the involved left scapula and shoulder (*arrows*) (Standard Uptake Value (SUV) 4.7; Note: typically normal soft tissue <1 SUV; normal bone marrow <3 SUV).

Differential Diagnosis

Osteomyelitis; metastatic disease; Ewing sarcoma (if younger patient); malignant fibrous histiocytoma, leukemia

Teaching Points

▶ Lymphoma is one of the round blue cell tumors. There are two types: Hodgkin's and non-Hodgkin's. Primary (<5%; typically non-Hodgkin's) or secondary . Invades via hematogenous or direct spread.

▶ Imaging features: (1) minimal cortical destruction in presence of extensive ST and marrow involvement or (2) permeative pattern of cortical bone with small cortical channels and (i) near-normal radiograph (particularly if primary and involves the knee) with little ST mass or (ii) destructive ossific lesion, periosteal reaction, and large ST mass (this case)

▶ Post-contrast studies demonstrate heterogeneous diffuse enhancement of a soft tissue component that often involves both intramedullary and extramedullary spaces.

▶ Whole-body MR or potentially whole-body diffusion weighted imaging can improve diagnostic accuracy for lymphomas that are FDG-avid and aid in management.

▶ Common locations—primary: long bones (particularly the knee); secondary: axial skeleton

Management

Image-guided biopsy is required for diagnosis. Whole-body PET-CT (in particular CT of the chest) and bone scan are typically required to assess for extent of disease and exclude metastatic disease. Presurgical treatment includes radiation or chemotherapy with postsurgical adjuvant chemotherapy.

Further Readings

Gu J, Chan T, Zhang J, Leung A, Kwong Y, Khong P. Original research: Whole body diffusion weighted imaging: the added value to whole body MRI at initial diagnosis of lymphoma. *AJR Am J Roentgenol* 2011;*197*:W384–W391.

Mengiardi B, Honegger H, Hodler J, Exner U, Csherhati M, Bruhlmann W. Original report: Primary lymphoma of bone: MRI and CT characteristics during and after successful treatment. *AJR Am J Roentgenol* 2005;*184*:185–192.

Case 43

History

- 80-year-old man with pain, swelling, and decreased range of motion of the right knee

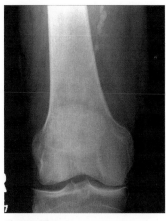

Figure 43.1

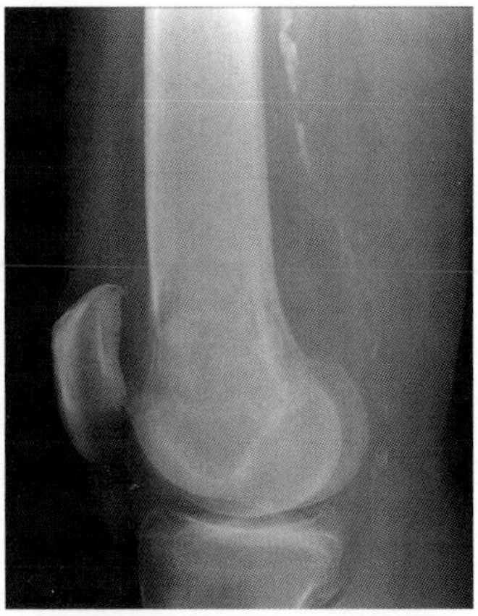

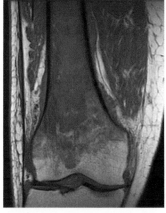

Figure 43.2

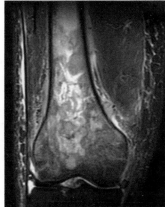

Figure 43.3

Figure 43.4

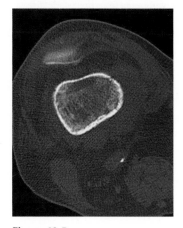

Figure 43.5

Case 43 Primary lymphoma of the knee

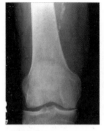

Figure 43.6

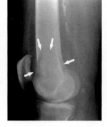

Figure 43.7

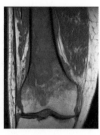

Figure 43.8

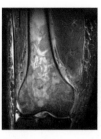

Figure 43.9

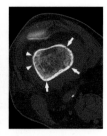

Figure 43.10

Findings

Figures 43.6 and 43.7 (AP and lateral radiographs of the right knee) demonstrate a moth-eaten/permeative lytic lesion of the distal right femur best seen on the lateral image (*white arrows*), with near-normal appearance on the AP view. Figures 43.8 and 43.9 (coronal T1 and STIR MR of the left knee) demonstrate abnormal low-signal-intensity (T1) and high-signal-intensity (STIR) intramedullary infiltrative disease of the distal femoral diametaphysis, including the epiphysis, with mild associated soft tissue extension. Figure 43.10 (axial CT of the distal right femur) shows minimal periosteal reaction (*arrowheads*), cortical lytic channels (*arrows*), and mixed intramedullary attenuation.

Differential Diagnosis

Lymphoma (primary more commonly than secondary); osteomyelitis; metastatic disease; Ewing sarcoma (if younger patient); leukemia, osteosarcoma (early)

Teaching Points

▸ Lymphoma is a round blue cell tumor. Two types: Hodgkin's and non-Hodgkin's. Primary type is less common (<5%; typically non Hodgkin's) than secondary type. Invades via hematogenous or direct spread.
▸ Locations—primary: long bones (particularly the knee, as in this case); secondary: axial skeleton
▸ Imaging features: (1) minimal cortical destruction in presence of soft tissue and marrow involvement or (2) permeative pattern of cortical bone destruction with small cortical channels best seen on CT and MRI with (i) near-normal radiograph (particularly if primary and involves the knee) with little soft tissue mass (as in this case) or (ii) destructive ossific lesion, periosteal reaction, and large soft tissue mass (more common in secondary type of lymphoma). (3) Presence of sequestrum may help differentiate primary lymphoma from metastatic disease.
▸ Post-contrast studies demonstrate heterogeneous diffuse enhancement of both intramedullary and extramedullary components. There is markedly abnormal uptake on Tc99 bone scans and PET-CT.

Management

Image-guided biopsy is required for diagnosis. Whole-body PET-CT and bone scan are typically required to assess for extent of disease and to exclude metastatic disease. Treatment includes chemotherapy with or without adjuvant radiation (83% 5-year survival rate in one study; therefore, diagnosis is important since lymphoma has a better survival rate than other potential differential diagnoses, such as metastatic disease or osteosarcoma).

Further Readings

Krishnan A, Shirkhoda A, Tehranzadeh J, Armin AR, Irwin R, Les K. Primary bone lymphoma—Radiographic MR imaging correlation. *Radiographics* 2003;*23*:1371–1383.
Mulligan ME, McRae GA, Murphey MD. Imaging features of primary lymphoma of bone. *AJR Am J Roentgenol* 1999;*173*:1691–1697.

History

▶ Diffuse bone pain

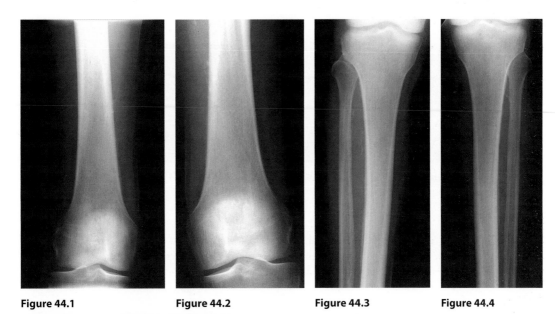

Figure 44.1   **Figure 44.2**   **Figure 44.3**   **Figure 44.4**

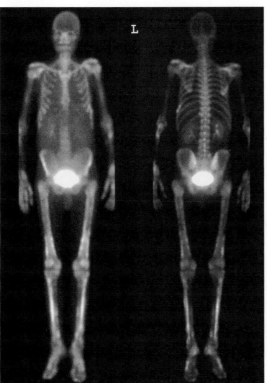

Figure 44.5

Figure 44.6

Case 44 Hypertrophic osteoarthropathy (lung cancer)

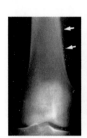 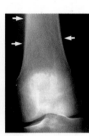 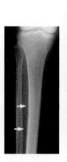 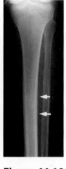 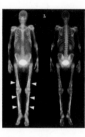 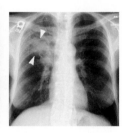

Figure 44.7   **Figure 44.8**   **Figure 44.9**   **Figure 44.10**   **Figure 44.11**   **Figure 44.12**

Findings

Figures 44.7 and 44.8 (AP radiographs of the distal femurs) and Figures 44.9 and 44.10 (proximal tibias) demonstrate subtle, linear periosteal new bone formation involving all four bones (*arrows*). Figure 44.11 (anterior and posterior views from whole-body radionuclide bone scan) reveal linear ("train track") areas of abnormal uptake in the long bones of the lower extremities (*arrowheads*). Figure 44.12 (PA view of the chest) demonstrates a large neoplasm in the right upper lobe (*arrowheads*).

Differential Diagnosis

Polyostotic periostitis: primary hypertrophic osteoarthropathy (pachydermo-periostosis); venous insufficiency; thyroid acropachy

Teaching Points

▶ Hypertrophic osteoarthropathy (HOA) is a disease of unknown pathophysiology that typically manifests with a clinical triad of arthritis-like symptoms, periostitis of the long bones, and clubbing of the fingers (although the latter is not always present).

▶ While the disease may occur in a primary form (also known as pachydermo-periostosis), 90% of cases are associated with an underlying malignancy, most commonly involving the lung.

▶ HOA may also occur with numerous nonneoplastic conditions such as cystic fibrosis, bacterial endocarditis, inflammatory bowel disease, and others.

▶ The primary radiographic feature of HOA is that of thin periosteal reaction typically involving the shafts of multiple long bones.

▶ Radionuclide bone scanning reveals abnormal, elongated ("train track") uptake, as seen in this case.

Management

Resection of the underlying tumor or lung transplantation (in the case of cystic fibrosis) may result in improvement. In addition to supportive analgesics, bisphosphonates have also been shown to provide relief in some patients.

Further Readings

Qingping Y, Altman RD, Brahn E. Periostitis and hypertrophic pulmonary osteoarthropathy: report of 2 cases and review of the literature. *Semin Arthritis Rheum* 2009;38:458–466.

History

► 40-year-old man with pain post injury to left forearm

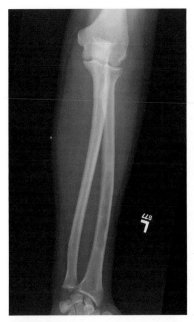

Figure 45.1

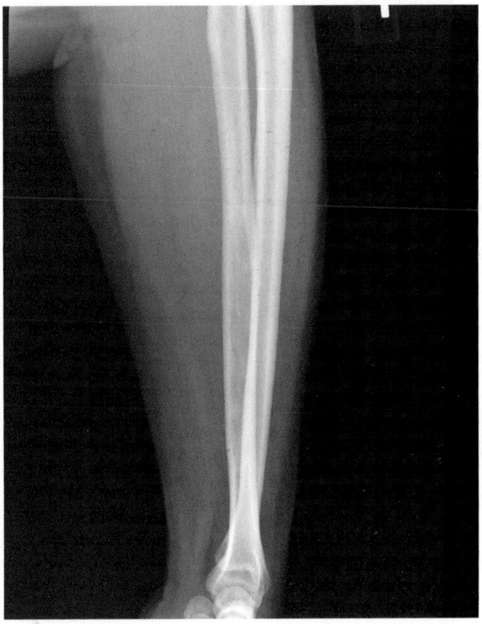

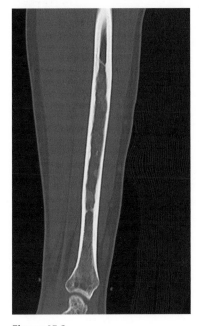

Figure 45.2

Figure 45.3

Case 45 Fibrous dysplasia

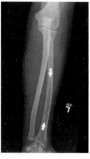 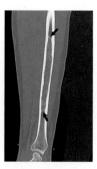

Figure 45.4   **Figure 45.5**   **Figure 45.6**

Findings

Figures 45.4 and 45.5 (AP/lateral left forearm radiographs) show an elongated, central intramedullary, hazy, well-defined lucency within the mid-distal ulnar diaphysis demonstrating mild endosteal scalloping and mild expansion (*white arrows*). The lesion is bordered by a zone of reactive sclerosis that is better appreciated on the sagittal CT (Fig. 45.6), as is the focally calcified or ossified matrix within the lesion giving rise to a "ground-glass" appearance (*black arrows*).

Differential Diagnosis

Chondromyxoid fibroma; neurofibromatosis; atypical metastatic disease (renal, thyroid, lung, breast) or myeloma, but these typically do not have a ground-glass appearance

Teaching Points

▶ Fibrous dysplasia is a skeletal developmental anomaly of bone-forming mesenchyme (osteoblasts fail to normally mature) associated with elevated serum alkaline phosphatase level. No sex predilection. Occurs between 10 and 70 years of age but commonly presents in the third or fourth decades.

▶ Monostotic (70% to 80%) and polyostotic (20% to 30%) varieties. The latter may be associated with endocrine dysfunction and cutaneous pigmentation (café-au-lait spots) (McCune-Albright syndrome).

▶ Common sites—monostotic: rib, femur, tibia, face, humerus; polyostotic: skull, face, pelvis, spine, shoulder. Diaphyseal location within long bones typical.

▶ Imaging: Ground-glass central intramedullary lucency, well-defined margins, zone of sclerosis and mild expansion with or without endosteal scalloping best seen on radiographs or CT. MR shows isointense/hypointense findings on T1-weighted images and heterogeneously hyperintense findings on T2-weighted images. The enhancement pattern is patchy central, rim, homogeneous, or a combination.

▶ Polyostotic involvement may be unilateral or asymmetric. Severe coxa vara abnormality of the proximal femoral neck and shaft may occur, known as the "shepherd's crook" deformity.

▶ Malignant transformation is rare (osteosarcoma or fibrosarcoma). Fractures may occur.

▶ Fibrous dysplasia (typically the polyostotic type) in association with intramuscular myxomas, is known as Mazabraud syndrome.

Management

Typically no treatment for asymptomatic lesions. If associated pain without trauma, evaluation for fracture, skeletal survey to assess for multiple lesions, or advanced imaging. If multiple lesions, assess for endocrine syndromes (hypophosphatemic rickets and osteomalacia and, particularly in females, McCune-Albright syndrome).

Further Readings

Kransdorf MJ, Moser RP, Gilkey FW. Fibrous dysplasia. *Radiographics* 1990;*10*(3):519–537.
Kumar R, Madewell J, Lindell M, Swischuk L. Fibrous lesions of bones. *Radiographics* 1990;*10*:237–256.
Shah ZK, Peh WC, Koh, WL, Shek TW. Magnetic resonance imaging of fibrous dysplasia. *Br J Radiol* 2005;*78*(936):1104–1115.

History

▶ 28-year-old woman with precocious sexual development and café-au-lait spots

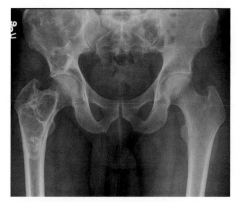

Figure 46.1

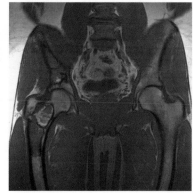

Figure 46.2

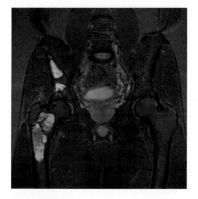

Figure 46.3

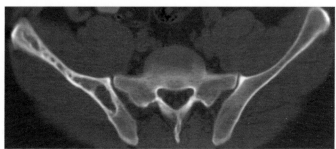

Figure 46.4

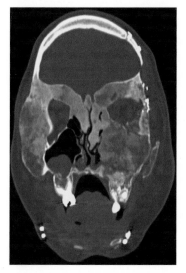

Figure 46.5

Case 46   McCune-Albright syndrome (polyostotic fibrous dysplasia)

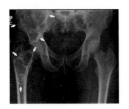 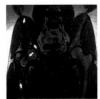 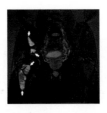 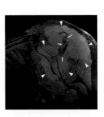 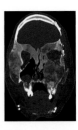

| Figure 46.6 | Figure 46.7 | Figure 46.8 | Figure 46.9 | Figure 46.10 |

Findings

Figure 46.6 (AP pelvis) shows well-defined central intramedullary lucent lesions of the proximal right femur and iliac bone with mild expansion (*white arrows on all images*). There is central isointensity on the coronal T1-weighted MR image (Fig. 46.7) with low-signal margins. Predominantly high signal intensity, with low-signal peripheral margins and mild central heterogeneity, is seen on STIR (Fig. 46.8). The axial pelvic CT (Fig. 46.9) and the coronal facial CT (Fig. 46.10) best depict intramedullary lucency, mild expansion, and ground-glass appearance, with peripheral sclerotic margins and facial expansion respectively.

Differential Diagnosis

Chondromyxoid fibroma; neurofibromatosis lesions; atypical metastatic disease (renal, thyroid, lung, breast) or myeloma, but these typically do not have ground-glass appearance or sclerotic margins; Paget's disease

Teaching Points

▸ Polyostotic fibrous dysplasia usually occurs in younger patients than does monostotic fibrous dysplasia (symptomatic before the age of 10 versus 10 to 70 years).
▸ It is a skeletal developmental anomaly of bone-forming mesenchyme (osteoblasts fail to mature normally) associated with elevated serum alkaline phosphatase levels.
▸ Triad of endocrine dysfunction, sexual precocity, and cutaneous pigmentation (café-au-lait spots that are fewer and more irregular in contour than those in neurofibromatosis)
▸ Sites: 50% involvement of the skull and face versus 10% to 25% in monostotic, followed by pelvis, spine, shoulder
▸ May be unilateral or asymmetric. Severe coxa vara abnormality of the proximal femoral neck and shaft leads to "shepherd's crook" deformity with higher risk of fractures.
▸ Imaging: Well-defined, often mildly expansile, intramedullary lucent lesion(s) demonstrating a "ground glass" appearance, with or without endosteal scalloping and areas of sclerosis. Predominantly outward calvarial expansion (convex) with typically undisturbed inner table. T1-weighted MR images show isointense/hypointense findings and T2-weighted images show heterogeneously hyperintense findings. The enhancement pattern is patchycentral, rim, homogeneous, or a combination.
▸ Malignant transformation is rare (osteosarcoma or fibrosarcoma). Mazabraud syndrome includes polyostotic fibrous dysplasia and intramuscular myxomas.

Management

No treatment for asymptomatic lesions, as many are quiescent at puberty. Lesions may be reactivated by pregnancy or estrogen therapy. If there is associated pain without trauma, a skeletal survey should be performed to assess for other lesions or advanced imaging to exclude fracture or rare malignancy. Assess for confirmation of the endocrine syndromes (hypophosphatemic rickets and osteomalacia and, particularly in females, McCune-Albright syndrome).

Further Readings

Kransdorf MJ, Moser RP, Gilkey, FW. Fibrous dysplasia. *Radiographics* 1990;*10*(3):519–537.
Kumar R, Madewell J, Lindell M, Swischuk L. Fibrous lesions of bones. *Radiographics* 1990;*10*:237–256.
Shah ZK, Peh WC, Koh, WL, Shek TW. Magnetic resonance imaging of fibrous dysplasia. *Br J Radiol* 2005;*78*(936):1104–1115.

History

► Unknown

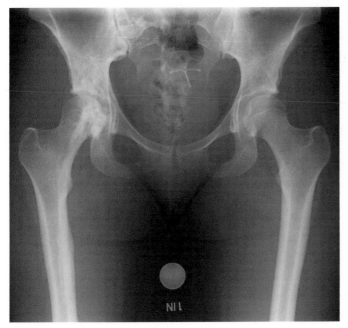

Figure 47.1

Case 47   Melorheostosis

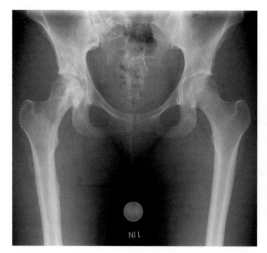

Figure 47.2

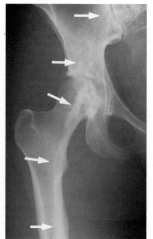

Figure 47.3

Findings

Figure 47.2 (AP radiograph of the pelvis) demonstrates asymmetric sclerosis involving the right iliac bone and femur. Figure 47.3 (coned-down frontal view) reveals to better advantage the patchy sclerosis within the medial iliac wing and its "flowing" appearance along the medial aspect of the proximal right femur, where there is marked, asymmetric cortical thickening (*arrows*).

Differential Diagnosis

Paget's disease

Teaching Points

▶ Melorheostosis is a sclerotic bone dysplasia that usually displays a distinctive radiographic appearance that includes prominent cortical hyperostosis, typically affecting one side of a bone, producing what's been described as a "dripping candle wax" appearance.

▶ The disease most commonly affects the lower extremities and often involves contiguous bones, as in this case.

▶ Radionuclide scanning reveals intensely increased uptake in the affected areas.

▶ CT clearly demonstrates the extent of the hyperostosis and degree of compromise of the medullary cavity.

▶ Areas of involvement are of homogeneously low intensity on all MR pulse sequences.

▶ In addition to the osseous involvement, mineralized and/or nonmineralized soft tissue masses may be present as well, and these benign lesions contain a mixture of chondroid, osseous, fibrolipomatous, and vascular elements.

Management

Although often asymptomatic, pain and other complications can occur. Nifedipine has been advocated for pain management, and surgery may be indicated for associated complications such as joint contracture, leg-length discrepancy, or articular involvement.

Further Readings

Judkiewicz AM, Murphey MD, Resnik CS, et al. Advanced imaging of melorheostosis with emphasis on MRI. *Skeletal Radiol* 2001;*30*:447–453.
Rozencwaig R, Wilson MR, McFarland GB Jr. Melorheostosis. *Am J Orthop* 1997;*26*:83–89.

Case 48

History

- 16-year-old boy with 1-month history of left hip and thigh pain worse at night, awaking him from sleep, and intermittent fevers. Tenderness to palpation.

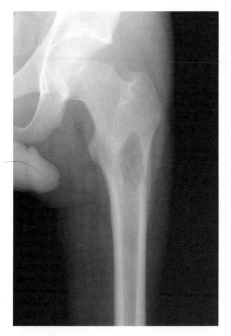

Figure 48.1

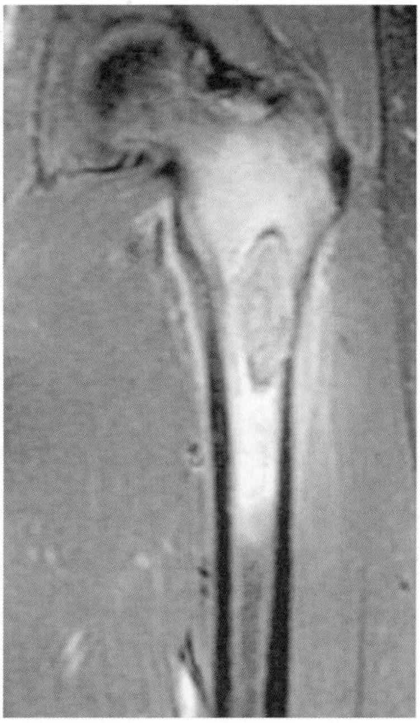

Figure 48.2

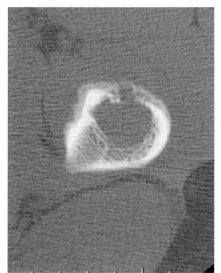

Figure 48.3

Case 48   Eosinophilic granuloma

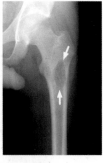
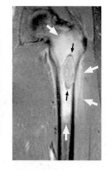
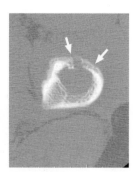

Figure 48.4   **Figure 48.5**   **Figure 48.6**

Findings

Figure 48.4 (AP radiograph of the left femur) shows a lytic intramedullary lesion within the subtrochanteric region (*white arrows*). MR demonstrated low signal on T1-weighted imaging with high signal intensity within the lesion and surrounding bone on T2-weighted imaging (not shown). Figure 48.5 (post gadolinium fat saturated T1-weighted coronal MR) demonstrates diffuse enhancement of the lesion, with mild peripheral predominance (*black arrows*), and additional enhancement of the adjacent bone marrow and surrounding soft tissues (*white arrows*). The margin, with mild endosteal erosion of cortex, is better appreciated on axial CT (Fig. 48.6). Tc99 bone scan showed marked uptake (not shown) without other lesions.

Differential Diagnosis

Osteomyelitis; Ewing sarcoma, lymphoma; fibrous dysplasia; chondromyxoid fibroma; atypical metastatic lesion (neuroblastoma)

Teaching Points

▸ Langerhans cell histiocytosis traditionally has encompassed three entities: eosinophilic granuloma (most common and mildest disease form with single or multiple lytic lesions, often with characteristic beveled edge), Hand Schuller Christian disease (triad of chronic ossific lesions, diabetes insipidus, and exophthalmos), and Letterer Siwe disease (acute rapid form with poor clinical prognosis with disseminated ossific lesions and visceral involvement).
▸ Pathology: Langerhans cells characterized by cytoplasmic inclusion bodies
▸ Clinical: Children, adolescents or young adults. Local pain, tenderness, swelling or mass, fever, and leukocytosis, but may be asymptomatic.
▸ Common sites: Skull, mandible, spine, ribs, and long bones (diaphyseal or metaphyseal > epiphyseal).
▸ Imaging: Solitary > multiple lesions. Well-defined lucent lesions with endosteal erosion of cortex and periosteal new bone formation. Often has a characteristic "beveled" appearance in skull lesions due to unequal destruction of the inner and outer tables of the vault and "button sequestrum" (radiodense focus in lytic cranial lesion). "Floating teeth" appearance in mandible.
▸ Complications: Pathologic fracture (ribs commonly). Vertebra plana (thoracic and lumbar predominance).

Management

Evaluate for pathologic fracture, particularly in rib lesions. Expansile lesions involving vertebral bodies and posterior elements can occur without significant collapse, although vertebra plana is common in the spine and advanced imaging may be useful. Skeletal survey should be done to evaluate for other lesions. Biopsy should be done to confirm benign eosinophilic granuloma versus potential osteomyelitis or lymphoma.

Further Readings

Azouz EM, Saigal G, Rodriquez Mm, Podda A. Langerhans' cell histiocytostis: pathology, imaging and treatment of skeletal involvement. *Pediatr Radiol* 2005;35(2):101–115.

Resnik D. *Diagnosis of bone and joint disorders*, 3rd ed., vol. 6. Philadelphia: Saunders, 1995.

History

▶ 35-year-old woman with right lower leg pain and swelling

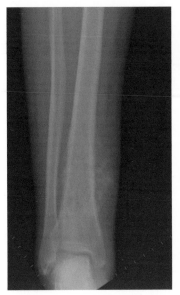

Figure 49.1

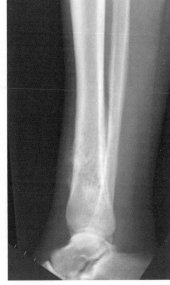

Figure 49.2

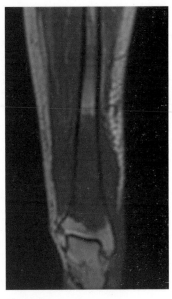

Figure 49.3

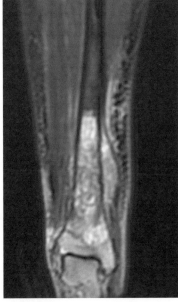

Figure 49.4

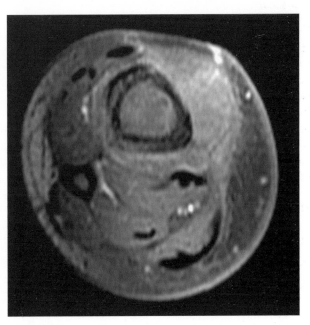

Figure 49.5

Case 49　Ewing sarcoma

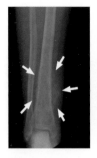
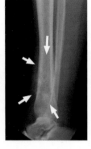
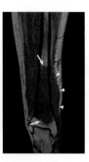
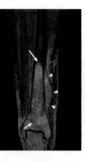
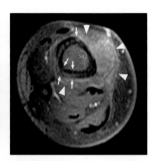

Figure 49.6　　**Figure 49.7**　　**Figure 49.8**　　**Figure 49.9**　　**Figure 49.10**

Findings

Figures 49.6 and 49.7 (radiographs) show moth-eaten/permeative, destructive distal tibial metadiaphyseal lesion with aggressive periosteal reaction and soft tissue swelling (*arrows*). Figures 49.8 and 49.9 (coronal T1-weighted and STIR MR) show low-signal (on T1-weighted image) and high-signal (STIR image) distal tibial lesion (*arrows*) with soft tissue component extending beyond cortex (*arrowheads*). Figure 49.10 (axial T2-weighted FS post-gadolinium MR image) shows multiple enhancing vascular cortical channels (*arrows*)with enhancing soft tissue (ST) tumor (*arrowheads*) extending from the intramedullary to extramedullary space.

Differential Diagnosis

Lymphoma/leukemia; osteosarcoma; osteomyelitis; fibrosarcoma

Teaching Points

▶ Ewing sarcoma is a small round blue cell tumor characterized by a permeative destructive bone pattern best visualized on CT/MR as small cortical vascular channels by which soft tissue tumor extends through bone.

▶ It is the second most common tumor in children, occurring in younger patients (3 to 25 years). It is the fourth most common primary bone tumor in adults, with metastasis more common in patients >40 years.

▶ Post-contrast studies demonstrate heterogeneous diffuse enhancement of a soft tissue component often involving both intramedullary and extramedullary spaces.

▶ Aggressive periosteal reaction (Codman's triangle, onionskin appearance, or sunburst pattern) is often present.

▶ Common locations: 60% of cases occur in long bones, typically metadiaphyseal not crossing the growth plate (femur > tibia > humerus). 40% occur in flat bones (pelvis and ribs).

▶ Presentation includes fever, increased leukocytosis, pain, and swelling. It may be confused with infection clinically.

Management

Image-guided biopsy is required for diagnosis. Metastasis is most common to the lung; chest radiograph/CT and bone scan are required to assess for extent of disease. Presurgical treatment includes radiation or chemotherapy with postsurgical adjuvant chemotherapy to reduce recurrence. New approaches include anti-angiogenic therapy.

Further Readings

Bernstein M, Kovar H, Paulussen M, Randall RL, Schuck A Teot LA, Juergens H. Ewing's sarcoma family of tumors: Current management. *Oncologist* 2006;*11*(5):503–519.

Kransdorf M, Smith SE. Lesions of unknown histogenesis: Langerhans cell histiocytosis and Ewing sarcoma. *Semin Musculoskelet Radiol* 2000;*4*(1):113–125.

Mar WA, Taljanovic MS, Bagatell R, Graham AR, Speer DP, Hunter TB, Rogers LF. Update on imaging and treatment of Ewing sarcoma family tumors: what the radiologist needs to know. *J Comput Assist Tomogr* 2008;*32*(1):108–118.

Case 50

History

- None

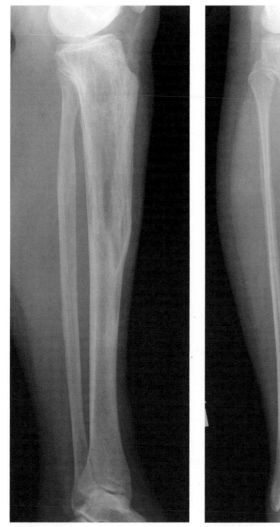

Figure 50.1

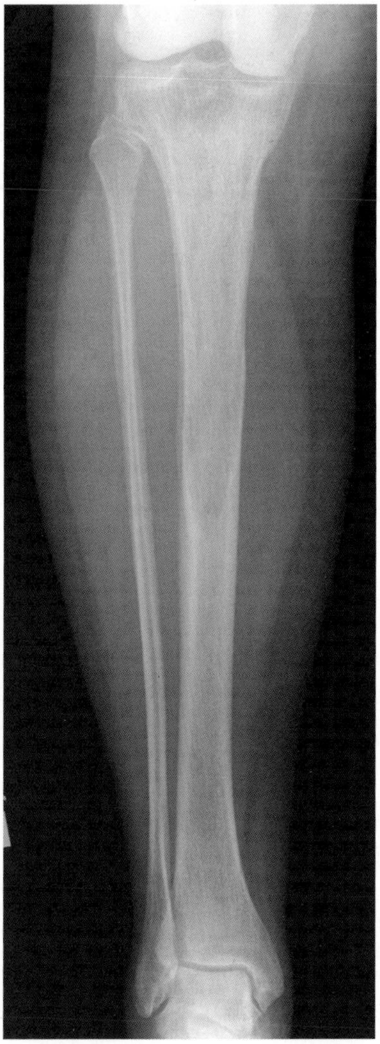

Figure 50.2

Case 50 Paget's disease

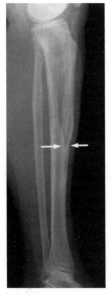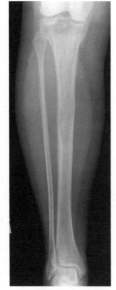

Figure 50.3　　　　**Figure 50.4**

Findings

Figures 50.3 and 50.4 (lateral and AP views of the lower leg) demonstrate mild expansion of the proximal tibia with mixed lytic and sclerotic changes and prominent coarsening of the trabeculae, findings consistent with Paget's disease. Note also the lytic, "blade of grass" appearance at the transition point between the normal and abnormal bone in Figure 50.3 (*arrows*).

Differential Diagnosis

None

Teaching Points

▸ Paget's disease is an idiopathic syndrome most commonly seen in patients >50, producing pain in approximately 30% of those affected.
▸ It can affect virtually any bone in the body but most commonly involves the pelvis and sacrum, spine, femur, and skull.
▸ It is typically divided into three phases—lytic, mixed, and sclerotic—with features of all three often present at the time of diagnosis.
▸ When it affects a long bone, it usually begins at one end and progresses to the other, with the interface between the advancing lytic changes and normal bone often forming a "blade of grass" appearance, as in this case. Other characteristic features include cortical thickening, coarsened trabeculae, and bone expansion.

Management

Bisphosphonates in patients with pain, markedly elevated bone alkaline phosphatase levels, and/or involvement in critical locations such as adjacent to nerve roots, joints, etc.

Further Readings

Colina M, LaCorte R, DeLeonardis F, Trotta F. Paget's disease of bone; a review. *Rheumatol Int* 2008;*28*:1069–1075.
Whitehouse RW. Paget's disease of bone. *Semin Musculoskelet Radiol* 2002;6:313–322.

History

▶ Palpable mass

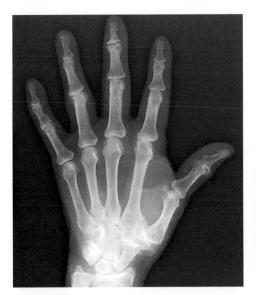

Figure 51.1

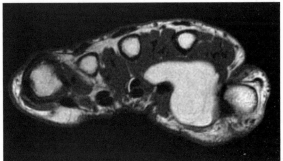

Figure 51.2

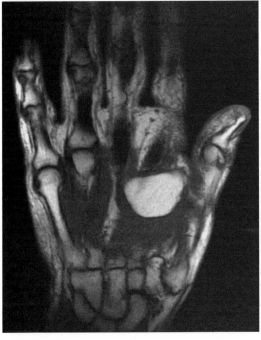

Figure 51.3

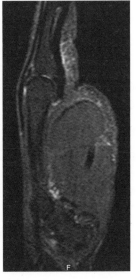

Figure 51.4

Case 51 Lipoma

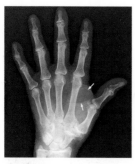

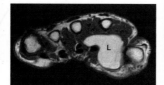

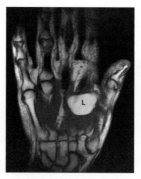

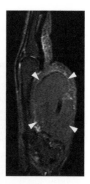

Figure 51.5   **Figure 51.6**   **Figure 51.7**   **Figure 51.8**

Findings

Figure 51.5 (AP view of the hand) reveals an ovoid lucency in the soft tissues of the hand (*arrows*) compatible with a fatty lesion. Axial (Fig. 51.6) and coronal (Fig. 51.7) T1-weighted MR images demonstrate a focal mass displaying homogeneous fatty signal intensity (L). Figure 51.8 (fat-saturated T2-weighted sagittal image) shows complete suppression of the signal from the lesion (*arrowheads*), confirming its fatty nature.

Differential Diagnosis

None. Atypical lipoma must be considered if thick or nodular non-fat signal intensity components are identified within the mass.

Teaching Points

▸ Lipomatous tumors lie along a spectrum from benign lipomas to high-grade liposarcomas.
▸ Benign lipomas are made up of mature adipose tissue and can be confidently diagnosed with MR imaging based on their homogeneous high signal on T1-weighted images that is completely suppressed on fat-saturated images. Thin low-signal septations and/or vessels are commonly seen within simple lipomas as well.
▸ Benign, intramuscular lipomas often appear quite infiltrative and demonstrate very irregular margins.
▸ Malignant lesions contain greater amounts of nonfatty tissue, and high-grade liposarcomas often contain little if any fat.

Management

Clinical and radiographic monitoring. Surgical therapy for painful lesions.

Further Readings

Gaskin CM, Helms CA. Lipomas, lipoma variants, and well-differentiated liposarcomas (atypical lipomas): results of MRI evaluations of 126 consecutive fatty masses. *AJR Am J Roentgenol.* 2004;*182*:733–739.
Wu JS, Hochman MG. Soft-tissue tumors and tumorlike lesions: a systematic imaging approach. *Radiology* 2009;*253*:297–316.

History

▸ 72-year-old man with palpable medial left thigh mass

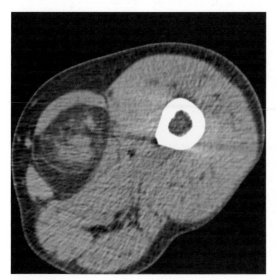

Figure 52.1

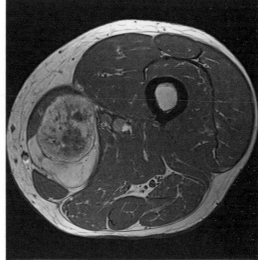

Figure 52.2

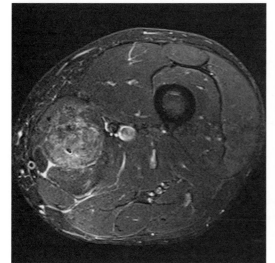

Figure 52.3

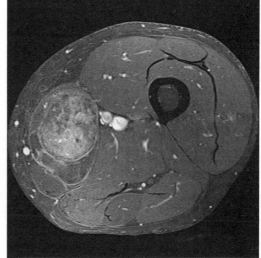

Figure 52.4

Case 52 Liposarcoma (dedifferentiated type)

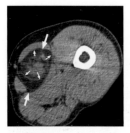

Figure 52.5

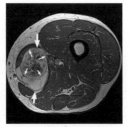

Figure 52.6

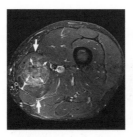

Figure 52.7

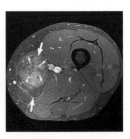

Figure 52.8

Findings

Axial CT (Fig. 52.5) and T1-weighted (Fig. 52.6), STIR (Fig. 52.7), and T1-weighted FS post-gadolinium (Fig. 52.8) MR images demonstrate a heterogeneous soft tissue mass (*large arrows*) within the medial left thigh abutting the posterior margin of the sartorius. Areas of predominantly fat are seen on CT and MR with a juxtaposed central anterior ovoid heterogeneous focal soft tissue nodular component (*small arrows*) (abnormal signal intensity and heterogeneous enhancement after intravenous administration of gadolinium). No abnormal mineralization is seen.

Differential Diagnosis

Fairly pathognomonic however could include: Myxoid tumors; fatty replacement of muscle; lAtypical ipoma

Teaching Points

▶ Liposarcoma is the second most common soft tissue tumor and tends to occur in the extremities (lower > upper 4:1).
▶ Imaging characteristics help differentiate liposarcoma from simple lipoma:
  1. Lack of homogeneous fatty tissue
  2. Thickened septations
  3. Presence of nonadipose soft tissue nodules
  4. Enhancement of soft tissue components, confirming nonadipose tissue
  5. Large size (>10 cm is suspicious for liposarcoma and should be followed)
▶ Typically seen in older patients, with pain and tenderness occurring in 10% to 15%.
▶ WHO classification of liposarcomas
  ▪ *Well differentiated* (most common type): Low-grade sarcoma that recurs locally, does not metastasize, and is considered atypical if superficial in location. Majority >75% fat. May have calcifications (10% to 15%). Good prognosis.
  ▪ *Dedifferentiated* (as in this case): Bimorphic lesion with high-grade pleomorphic sarcoma of nonadipose cells focal and juxtaposed with low-grade well-differentiated liposarcoma
  ▪ *Myxoid:* Intermediate grade may coexist with hypercellular form high grade. Predilection for extrapulmonary metastases.
  ▪ *Pleomorphic:* High grade and least common type

Management

Advanced imaging (CT/MR) distinguishes fat from nonadipose components. Contrast differentiates soft tissue components and extent of lesion. Image-guided biopsy of the nonadipose component is needed for diagnosis. CT of the chest/abdomen is used to evaluate for metastatic disease in subtypes other than well-differentiated liposarcoma.

Further Readings

Kransdorf MJ, Murphey MD. *Lipomatous tumors. In Imaging of Soft Tissue Tumors*, 2nd ed. Philadelphia: Lippincott Williams and Wilkins, 2006:125–149.
Murphey MD, Arcara LK, Fanburg-Smith J. Imaging of musculoskeletal liposarcoma with radiologic–pathologic correlation. *Radiographics* 2005;25;1371–1395.

History

▶ 29-year-old man with palpable medial left thigh mass

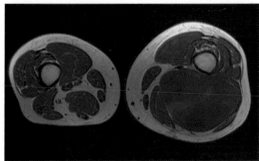

Figure 53.1

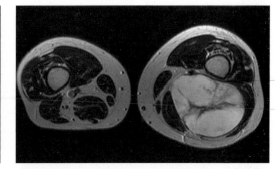

Figure 53.2

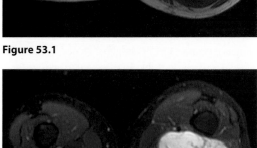

Figure 53.3

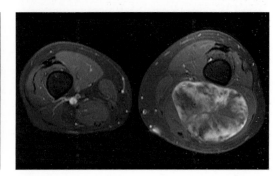

Figure 53.4

Case 53 Myxoid liposarcoma

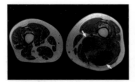
Figure 53.5

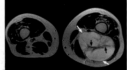
Figure 53.6

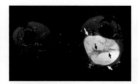
Figure 53.7

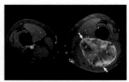
Figure 53.8

Findings

MR images of the left thigh (axial T1-weighted, Fig. 53.5; T2-weighted, Fig. 53.6; STIR, Fig. 53.7) demonstrate a large nonspecific heterogeneous soft tissue mass of the posteromedial thigh/popliteal fossa (*white arrows*). It is of predominantly low signal intensity on the T1-weighted image and high signal intensity on the T2-weighted image, with internal areas of high (T1) and intermediate (T2, STIR) signal intensity (*black arrows*) following the imaging characteristics of fat (fat <25% of the volume of the mass). Figure 53.8 (T1-weighted FS post-gadolinium image) demonstrates diffuse heterogeneous enhancement of solid portions of the mass sparing the infiltrative fatty areas (*F*). Extrapulmonary metastases were present at time of presentation (not shown).

Differential Diagnosis

Myxoid tumors; fatty replacement of muscle; lipoma or intramuscular myxoma

Teaching Points

▶ Liposarcoma is the second most common soft tissue tumor and tends to occur in the extremities (lower > upper 4:1).
▶ Imaging characteristics help differentiate liposarcoma from simple lipoma:
  1. Lack of homogeneous fatty tissue
  2. Thickened septations
  3. Presence of nonadipose soft tissue nodules
  4. Enhancement of soft tissue components, confirming nonadipose tissue
  5. Large size (>10 cm is suspicious for liposarcoma and should be followed)
▶ Typically seen in older patients; pain and tenderness in 10% to 15%
▶ WHO classification of liposarcomas
  ▪ *Well differentiated* (most common type): Low-grade sarcoma that recurs locally, does not metastasize, and is considered atypical if superficial in location. Majority >75% fat. May have calcifications (10% to 15%). Good prognosis.
  ▪ *Dedifferentiated*: Bimorphic lesion with high-grade pleomorphic sarcoma of nonadipose cells focal and juxtaposed with low-grade well-differentiated liposarcoma
  ▪ *Myxoid* (this case): Intermediate grade may coexist with hypercellular form high grade. Predilection for extrapulmonary metastases.
  ▪ *Pleomorphic:* High grade and least common type

Management

Advanced imaging (CT/MR) distinguishes fat from nonadipose components. Contrast differentiates soft tissue components and extent of lesion. Image-guided biopsy of the nonadipose component is needed for diagnosis. CT of the chest/abdomen is used to evaluate for metastatic disease in subtypes other than well-differentiated liposarcoma.

Further Readings

Kransdorf MJ, Murphey MD. Lipomatous t*umors. In Imaging of Soft Tissue Tumors*, 2nd ed. Philadelphia: Lippincott Williams and Wilkins, 2006:125–149.
Murphey MD, Arcara LK, Fanburg-Smith J. Imaging of musculoskeletal liposarcoma with radiologic–pathologic correlation. *Radiographics* 2005;1371–1395.

History

► 20-year-old male with palpable right dorsal ankle mass

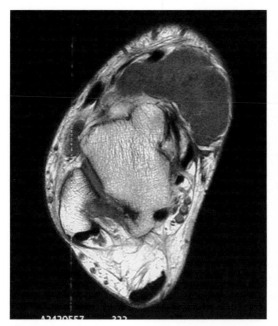

Figure 54.1

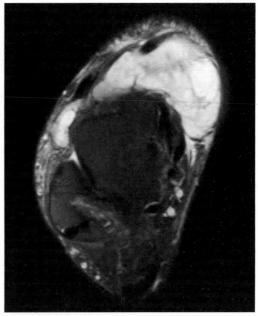

Figure 54.2

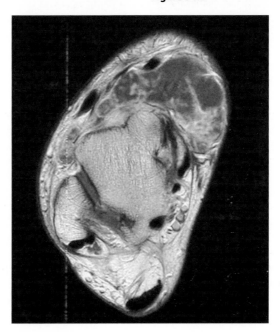

Figure 54.3

Case 54 Synovial sarcoma

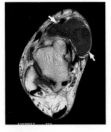
Figure 54.4

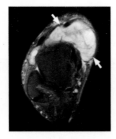
Figure 54.5

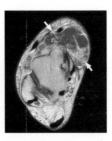
Figure 54.6

Findings

Ankle radiographs (not shown) showed nonspecific soft tissue swelling over the dorsal medial ankle without calcification. Axial T1-weighted (Fig. 54.4) and T2-weighted fat-saturated (Fig. 54.5) MR images demonstrate a lobulated, elongated, well-defined dorsal medial soft tissue mass (intermediate low/heterogeneous signal T1; bright heterogeneous signal T2) without definite fat or connection to the ankle joint (*white arrows*). Axial T1-weighted post-gadolinium MR image (Fig. 54.6) confirms a heterogeneously enhancing soft tissue mass (*white arrows*), excluding a simple ganglion.

Differential Diagnosis

MR images are nonspecific however the differential diagnosis could include: ganglion or synovial cyst (if the lesion had showed peripheral thin enhancement); soft tissue metastasis or fluid collection on initial images (not on post-contrast images); well-differentiated liposarcoma

Teaching Points

▶ Synovial sarcoma is a soft tissue malignancy that occurs in younger patients (15 to 40 years of age). It represents 5% to 10% of all sarcomas, originates from undifferentiated mesenchymal tissue, not synovium, and occurs around joints but not from joints (with the exception of a rare intra-articular variant).
▶ 80% to 90% occur within the extremities (60% to 70% in lower limbs).
▶ Three histologic types: monophasic, biphasic, and poorly differentiated.
▶ Common clinical presentation is a palpable mass with pain or sensory symptoms. Slow growth and a well-defined appearance on imaging may lead to confusion with a benign process.
▶ 30% may have calcifications (often in the periphery) best seen on CT or radiographs, with 10% showing periosteal reaction or bone involvement. Juxta-articular osteopenia may be present.
▶ MR demonstrates a nonspecific, inhomogeneous, usually well-defined mass that may mimic a benign-appearing mass, with fluid–fluid levels in 25%, prior hemorrhage in 40%, and "triple signal" intensity appearance on T2-weighted MR due to cystic and solid elements.
▶ Heterogeneous enhancement, prominence on angiography and increased activity on bone scan blood flow and pool images reflect marked vascularity.
▶ Metastatic disease is present in 80%; 25% have metastases on presentation (lung > lymph nodes > bone).

Management

Treatment is wide surgical excision, with radical resection and radiation therapy utilized for high-grade lesions and chemotherapy for metastatic disease or residual disease. Radiologic monitoring is required after treatment as recurrence rate is high (70% to 80%). 5-year survival rate is 25% to 61%. Lesions with calcifications have been shown to have a better prognosis.

Further Readings:

Jones BC, Sundaram M, Kransdorf MJ. Synovial sarcoma: MR imaging findings in 34 patients. *AJR Am J Roentgenol* 1993;*161*:827–883.
Murphey MD, Gibson M, Jennings BT, Crespo-Rodriquez A, Fanburg-Smith J, Gajewaki D. Imaging of synovial sarcoma with radiologic-pathologic correlation. *Radiographics* 2006;*26*:1543–1565.

History

▶ Mass

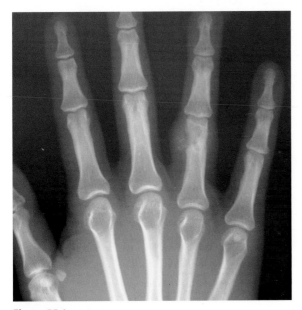

Figure 55.1

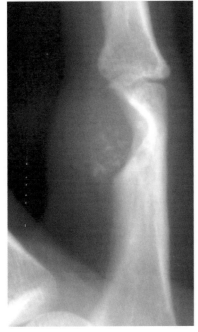

Figure 55.2

Case 55 Periosteal chondroma

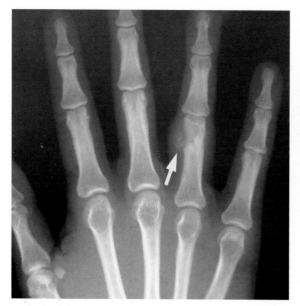

Figure 55.3

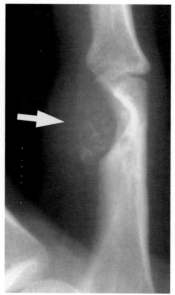

Figure 55.4

Findings

AP view of the hand (Fig. 55.3) and coned-down lateral view of the ring finger (Fig. 55.4) demonstrate a soft tissue mass containing punctate calcifications (*arrow*) along the radial/volar aspect of the finger producing smooth erosion of the underlying bone.

Differential Diagnosis

Other surface lesions such as periosteal chondrosarcoma, periosteal osteosarcoma, and high-grade surface osteosarcoma, but in this case the features are essentially pathognomonic.

Teaching Points

▶ Periosteal chondroma is a benign lesion involving the surface of the bone that often presents as a palpable mass.
▶ The most common sites of involvement include the phalanges of the hands and feet and the proximal humerus.
▶ The radiographic appearance of this lesion is usually diagnostic: a surface mass containing variable amounts of punctate calcification with prominent scalloping of the underlying bone, usually with a sclerotic margin.

Management

Marginal excision or curettage. Incomplete excision may result in a local recurrence.

Further Readings

Yildirim C, Unay K, Rodop O, Gamsizkan M. Periosteal chondroma that presented as a subcutaneous mass in the ring finger. *J Plast Surg Hand Surg* 2011;45:117–120.

History

▶ 45-year-old woman with palpable painless mass of the left knee

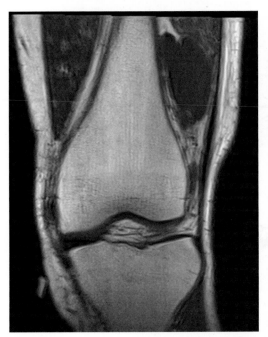

Figure 56.1

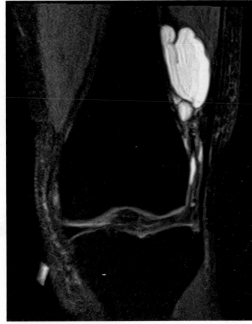

Figure 56.2

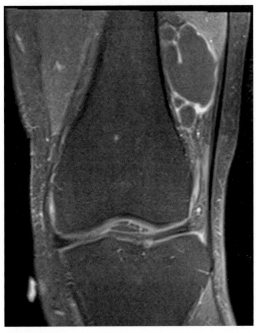

Figure 56.3

Case 56 Ganglion cyst

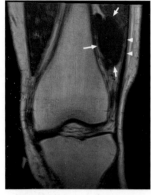

Figure 56.4

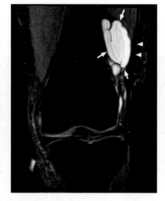

Figure 56.5

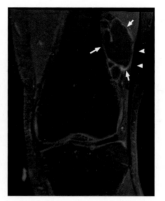

Figure 56.6

Findings

Figure 56.4 (coronal T1-weighted MR image) demonstrates a well-defined, lobulated homogeneous collection (*white arrows all images*) isointense to muscle located within the soft tissues deep to the iliotibial band (*arrowheads all images*) and adjacent to the distal lateral femur. Figure 56.5 (coronal T2-weighted FS MR image) shows diffuse homogeneous high signal intensity within the well-defined collection. Figure 56.6 (coronal T1-weighted FS MR post-gadolinium image) confirms a lobulated, well-defined homogeneous cystic fluid collection with a thin peripheral rim of enhancement without enhancement or nodularity within the remainder of the collection.

Differential Diagnosis

Pathognomic but could include: synovial cyst; bursa; infected fluid collection; rare cystic sarcoma

Teaching Points

▶ Ganglion cysts are common soft tissue masses, but they are not considered to be true soft tissue tumors.
▶ Common locations are the hands, wrist, and feet. They can arise from joint capsules, bursae, ligaments, tendons, and subchondral bone. Some may have communication with the joint, making it difficult to differentiate from periarticular cysts.
▶ Imaging follows underlying tissue pathology: well-defined, round or ovoid, homogeneous, lobulated fluid collection with a thin spindle cell rim without a synovial lining in close proximity to a joint or tendon. The spindle cell rim contributes to the characteristic rim of peripheral enhancement on CT or MR that helps distinguish this cystic lesion from solid lesions. Central homogeneous fluid of a ganglion cyst is typically of intermediate/low signal intensity (T1); bright (T2); intermediate/low (T1 FS). Cysts may occasionally be hyperintense to muscle on T1-weighted imaging due to higher proteinaceous content.
▶ US: anechoic or hypoechoic cystic structure with a hyperechoic rim
▶ Typically there are no findings on radiographs, but larger lesions can give rise to chronic remodeling of bone.

Management

No treatment is needed unless there is secondary nerve or vascular compression or for cosmetic reasons. They can be aspirated or injected with steroid under US but typically recur.

Further Readings

Beaman FD, Petersen JJ. MR imaging of cysts, ganglia and bursae about the knee. *Radiol Clin North Am* 2007;*45*(6):969–982.
Wu JS, Hochman MG. Soft tissue tumors and tumorlike lesions: a systematic imaging approach. *Radiology* 2009;*253*:297–316.

History

▶ 16-year-old with painless palpable mass of the dorsal foot

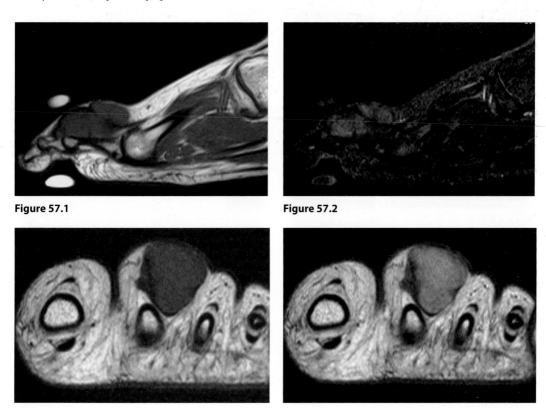

Figure 57.1

Figure 57.2

Figure 57.3

Figure 57.4

Case 57   Giant cell tumor of tendon sheath

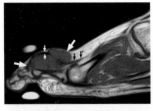

Figure 57.5

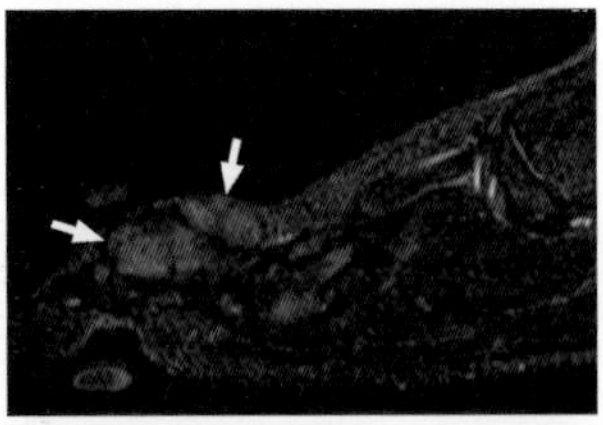

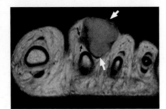

Figure 57.6

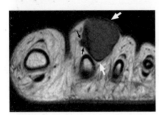

Figure 57.7

Figure 57.8

Findings

Figures 57.5 and 57.6 (Sagittal T1 and STIR) and Figures 57.7 and 57.8 (Coronal T1 and T1 post gadolinium) MR images demonstrate a solid, well-defined, smooth soft tissue mass (*white arrows all images*) arising from the second extensor tendon sheath of the foot (*small white and black arrows*). The lesion demonstrates homogeneous low/intermediate signal intensity on both T1 and STIR sequences with diffuse enhancement after contrast administration. No peripheral fluid or edema is present. There is no bone involvement.

Differential Diagnosis

Foreign body reaction (chronic); fibroma of the tendon sheath

Teaching Points

▶ Giant cell tumor of the tendon sheath (GCTTS) is the focal solid localized form of pigmented villonodular synovitis (PVNS), with characteristic low/intermediate signal intensity on all MR sequences due to hemosiderin/inflammatory material and may show diffuse enhancement.

▶ These tumors typically arise from the tendon sheath but can arise from the synovium.

▶ These tumors are more commonly seen in the digits of the hands (particularly the PIP joints), than the feet,(plantar involvement most common), but they can occur at any tendon site.

▶ 20% of patients present with chronic pressure erosions of adjacent bone, which can be a risk factor for recurrence.

▶ This is the second most common benign hand tumor (ganglion is the first).

▶ It is difficult to differentiate from a fibroma of the tendon sheath, although a fibroma typically does not enhance.

Management

Surgical removal, with recurrence noted in 10% to 20%. If cortical erosion is present, cortical removal is recommended to avoid recurrence.

Further Readings

Kransdorf M, Murphey M. *Synovial tumors. In Imaging of Soft Tissue Tumors*, 2nd ed. Philadelphia: Lippincott Williams and Wilkins, 2006: 381–436.

Murphey M, Rhee J, Lewis R, Fanburg-Smith J, Flemming D, Walker E. From the Archives of the AFIP: Pigmented villonodular synovitis: Radiologic–pathologic correlation. *Radiographics* 2008;28:1493–1518.

History

▶ Forearm mass

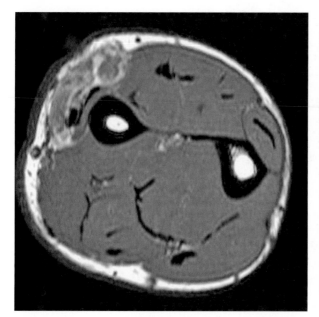

Figure 58.1

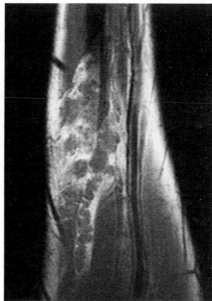

Figure 58.2

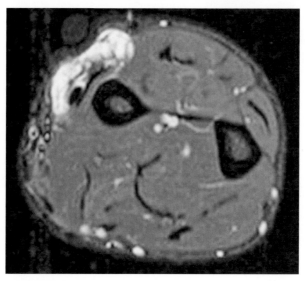

Figure 58.3

Case 58   Soft tissue hemangioma

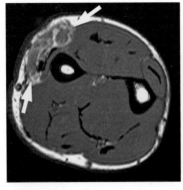

Figure 58.4

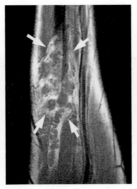

Figure 58.5

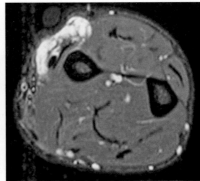

Figure 58.6

Findings

Figure 58.4 (axial T1-weighted image at the level of the mid-forearm) demonstrates a heterogeneous mass along the radial aspect of the forearm, involving the extensor carpi radialis brevis muscle (*arrows*). Figure 58.5 (sagittal T1-weighted image at that same level) reveals extensive high-signal-intensity fat between the intermediate-signal-intensity lobules of the mass (*arrows*). Figure 58.6 (axial STIR image) shows high signal intensity throughout the lobular mass with thin low-signal septa.

Differential Diagnosis

None

Teaching Points

▶ Soft tissue hemangiomas are most commonly found in children but may be discovered at any age.
▶ The lesion may be suspected on radiographs when calcified phleboliths are identified within a mass.
▶ The MR imaging appearance of a hemangioma is usually quite characteristic:
  – Blood-filled cavities that compose the lesion appear as multiple lobules that demonstrate markedly increased signal on fat-saturated T2-weighted images.
  – Fat is usually found among the lobules and is identified by its high signal intensity on T1-weighted images.
  – High-flow feeding or draining vessels will demonstrate signal voids within their lumen.

Management

Depending on the clinical situation, embolization and/or surgical resection may be indicated.

Further Readings

Papp DE, Khanna AJ, McCarthy EF, Carrino JA, Farber AJ, Frassica FJ. Magnetic resonance imaging of soft-tissue tumors: determinate and indeterminate lesions. *J Bone Joint Surg Am* 2007;89(Suppl 3):103–115.
Wu JS, Hochman MG. Soft-tissue tumors and tumorlike lesions: a systematic imaging approach. *Radiology* 2009;253:297–316.

History

▶ 11-year-old boy with mass at elbow

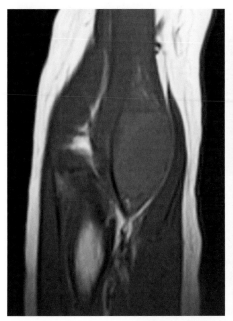

Figure 59.1

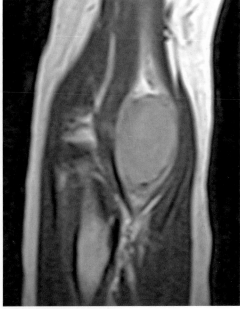

Figure 59.2

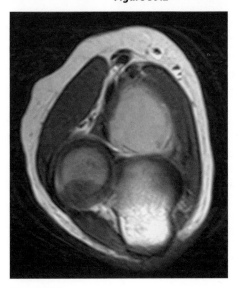

Figure 59.3

Case 59 Synovial sarcoma

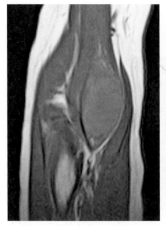

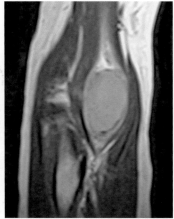

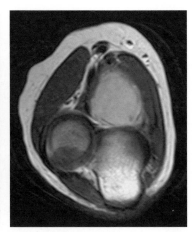

Figure 59.4 **Figure 59.5** **Figure 59.6**

Findings

Figure 59.4 (coronal T1-weighted image of the elbow) reveals an ovoid, smoothly marginated mass of intermediate signal intensity displacing the adjacent muscles. Coronal (Fig. 59.5) and axial (Fig. 59.6) T2-weighted images demonstrate relatively homogeneous slightly increased signal intensity within the mass as well as a few septations. Again, the mass displays smooth margins and appears to displace rather than invade the adjacent muscles.

Differential Diagnosis

The MR appearance is nonspecific and requires a broad differential diagnosis that includes both benign and malignant entities.

Teaching Points

▸ MR imaging is a powerful tool for evaluating a soft tissue mass since it provides not only a superb demonstration of its appearance and extent, but also a specific diagnosis in the case of lesions such as lipoma, ganglion cyst, giant cell tumor of the tendon sheath, hemangioma, etc.

▸ A majority of soft tissue lesions, however, do not demonstrate pathognomonic imaging features and must be considered "indeterminate" in nature.

▸ Depending on the clinical findings, biopsy should be strongly considered for most indeterminate lesions since many malignant entities will display a very nonaggressive appearance, as in this case.

Management

Ultimate management will depend upon biopsy results.

Further Readings

Wu JS, Hochman MG. Soft-tissue tumors and tumorlike lesions: a systematic imaging approach. *Radiology* 2009;*253*:297–316.

History

▸ 34-year-old woman with a palpable, firm, painless mass of the left shoulder

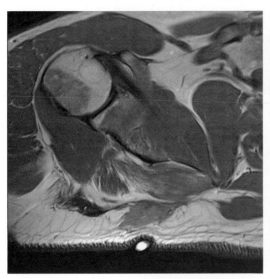

Figure 60.1

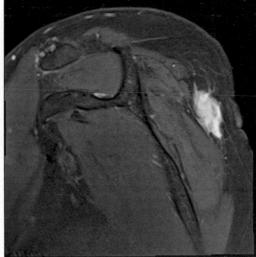

Figure 60.2

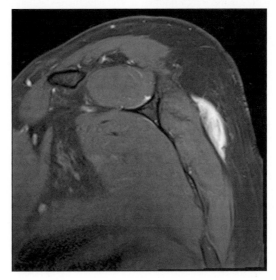

Figure 60.3

Case 60 Desmoid tumor (malignant-appearing benign lesion)

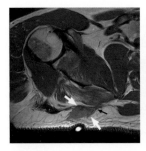 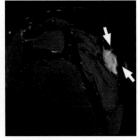 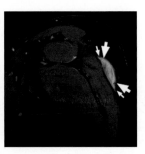

Figure 60.4   **Figure 60.5**   **Figure 60.6**

Findings

Figure 60.4 (axial PD MR image of the left shoulder) depicts a solitary oval intermediate-signal-intensity soft tissue lesion with spiculated, irregular, poorly circumscribed margins (*white arrows all images*) abutting the deep subcutaneous fascia with a "fascial tail" (*small arrows on all images*). Figure 60.5 (sagittal T1-weighted FS post-gadolinium MR image) confirms the deep subcutaneous soft tissue lesion abutting the fascia with some enhancement and irregular margins. Figure 60.6 (sagittal T1-weighted FS post-gadolinium image more posterior) demonstrates the lesion to be smooth and elongated, with superior and inferior fascial tails. No surrounding edema is present.

Differential Diagnosis

Foreign body reaction; metastatic disease (rare); nodular fasciitis; pigmented villonodular synovitis (low signal material); malignant fibrous histiocytoma; synovial sarcoma (nonspecific)

Teaching Points

▶ Desmoid-type fibromatosis refers to all extra-abdominal, abdominal, and intra-abdominal fibromatosis affecting the fascia, septa, and aponeuroses between muscles.

▶ There are superficial and deep types (deep are less common), and they are typically solitary, although synchronous lesions are present in 5% to 15%.

▶ Desmoid tumors are typically seen in young adults (peak age 25 to 35 years), they are considered benign, and they occur more frequently in women.

▶ Locations: shoulder/upper arm (28%); chest wall, paraspinal, thigh, head/neck (more aggressive), knee, buttock/hip, lower leg, forearm

▶ Radiographs are typically normal. MR (best), US (to assess vascularity), and CT are useful.

▶ Desmoid tumors may have irregular margins (as in this case) or smooth margins and have variable intensity or density based on the amount of fibrosis, which is commonly of low signal intensity on all sequences. Avid enhancement is due to the cellular component of these lesions.

▶ A characteristic "fascial tail," as in this case, should lead one to a desmoid diagnosis.

▶ There is no malignant potential, but desmoid tumors recur locally, so it is important to resect the entire fascial tail.

Management

Wide surgical resection is the treatment of choice (must excise entire lesion and tails). However, adjuvant radiation is also performed in many cases or is given as the only therapy in lesions too large to resect. Chemotherapy has been used successfully in some aggressive cases.

Further Readings

Dinauer PA, Brixey CJ, Moncur JT, Fanburg-Smith JC, Murphey M. Pathologic and MR imaging features of benign fibrous soft tissues tumors in adults. *Radiographics* 2007;27(1):173–187.

Murphey M, Kransdorf MJ. Benign fibrous and fibrohistiocystic tumors. In *Imaging of Soft Tissue Tumors*, 2nd ed. Philadelphia: Lippincott Williams and Wilkins, 2006:224–231.

History

▶ 27-year-old woman with intermittent focal pain, tenderness, and swelling of the right second intermetatarsal interspace. Pain during "squeeze test" of the second intermetatarsal space and positive Mulder click sign.

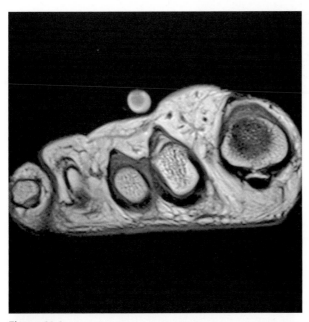

Figure 61.1

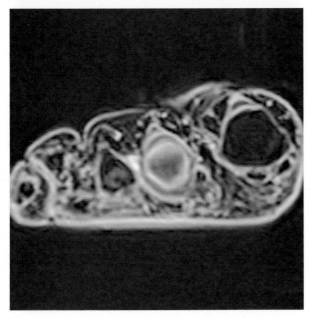

Figure 61.2

Case 61 Morton neuroma

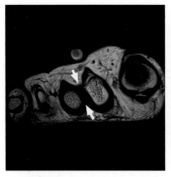

Figure 61.3

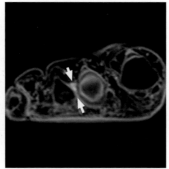

Figure 61.4

Findings

Coronal T1-weighted (Fig. 61.3) and VIBE fat-saturated post-gadolinium (Fig. 61.4) MR images of the right foot depict an oval, 4-mm, low-signal-intensity focus within the mid-second intermetatarsal interspace demonstrating homogeneous bright enhancement (*white arrows*). There is mild dorsal and plantar subcutaneous edema without bone marrow or cortical abnormality.

Differential Diagnosis

Intermetatarsal fluid; fibroma; foreign body reaction or granuloma (less likely)

Teaching Points

▶ Morton neuroma represents focal perineural fibrosis about a digital nerve (typically plantar but can be mid or dorsal), most commonly between the third and fourth metatarsal heads, followed by the second intermetatarsal interspace.

▶ Morton neuroma presents with intermittent pain and tingling at the site.

▶ There is a marked (18:1) female predilection (due to wearing of high heels).

▶ The Mulder sign is an audible click when metatarsal heads are squeezed together at the site of pain.

▶ Morton neuroma is not visible on radiographs and is best diagnosed on MR coronal T1-weighted images (low/intermediate-signal-intensity round/oval soft tissue mass) and T2-weighted images (signal intensity less than that of fat, likely reflecting high collagen content). Fat-saturated sequences help differentiate the lesion from surrounding tissues. Most tend to enhance diffusely and avidly.

Management

If not well seen on traditional MR, Weishaupt et al. describe improved visualization in the prone position due to dependence of the lesion. Treatment is typically conservative modification of footwear. Neurolysis, ultrasound-guided steroid injection, ultrasound therapy, and surgical release of the transverse metatarsal ligament for decompression have proven useful in refractory cases. Definitive treatment is surgical resection with a 10% incidence of traumatic neuroma.

Further Readings

Bencardino J, Rosenberg Z, Beltran J, Liu Z, Marty-Delfaut E. Morton's neuroma: is it always symptomatic? *AJR* Am J Roentgenol 2000;*175*;649–653.

Murphey MD, Smith S, Smith SE, Kransdorf M, Temple T. Imaging of musculoskeletal neurogenic tumors: radiologic–pathologic correlation. *Radiographics* 1999;*19*:1253–1280.

Weishaupt D, Treiber K, Kundert HP, Zollinger H, Vienne P, Hodler J, Willman J, Marincek B, Zanetti M. Morton neuroma: MR imaging in prone, supine, and upright weight-bearing body positions. *Radiology* 2003;*226*:849–856.

History

► Palpable plantar mass

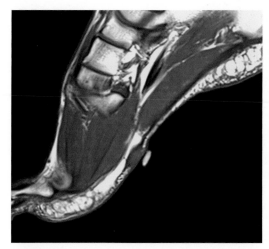

Figure 62.1

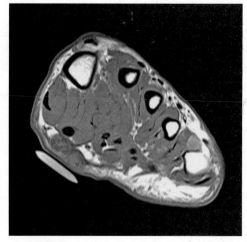

Figure 62.2

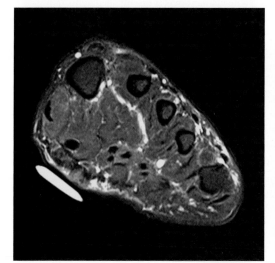

Figure 62.3

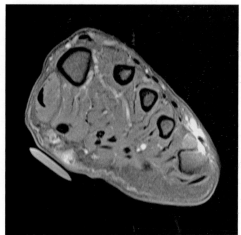

Figure 62.4

Case 62   Plantar fibroma

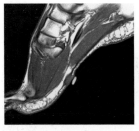

Figure 62.5

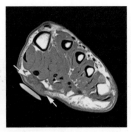

Figure 62.6

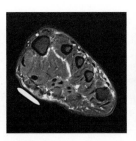

Figure 62.7

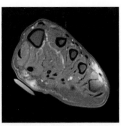

Figure 62.8

Findings

Figures 62.5 (sagittal) and 62.6 (short axis T1-weighted images) demonstrate a small nodular mass of intermediate signal intensity beneath the skin marker within the plantar fascia (*arrows*). The mass demonstrates relatively low signal intensity on a short axis fat-saturated T2-weighted image (Fig. 62.7) and prominent enhancement on a short axis fat-saturated T1-weighted image after the intravenous administration of gadolinium (Fig. 62.8).

Differential Diagnosis

Giant cell tumor of the tendon sheath (but the association with the plantar fascia is essentially diagnostic)

Teaching Points

▶ Plantar fibromatosis is a benign disorder of fibroblastic proliferation within the plantar aponeurosis and is one of the superficial fibromatoses that include Dupuytren's contracture in the hand.

▶ The disease results in one or more (usually palpable) masses along the sole of the foot that most typically involve the central band of the plantar aponeurosis. These are multiple in 30% of cases and bilateral in 20% to 50% of cases.

▶ Ultrasound reveals hypoechoic or heterogeneous nodules adjacent to the plantar aponeurosis, with most demonstrating increased vascularity with color Doppler imaging.

▶ Because of their fibrous nature, these lesions will typically demonstrate intermediate to low signal intensity on both T1- and T2-weighted images, a feature that may make lesion detection challenging. The vast majority of lesions, however, will enhance after contrast administration, so post-contrast imaging should be a part of any MR protocol when this disorder is suspected.

Management

Typically, management is conservative (footwear modification, etc.), with surgery reserved for large or painful lesions due to a high rate of postoperative recurrence.

Further Readings

Murphey MD, Ruble CM, Tyszko SM, Zbohniewicz AM, Potter BK, Miettinen M. Musculoskeletal fibromatoses: radiologic–pathologic correlation. *Radiographics*. 2009;29:2143–2173.

History

▶ 32-year-old man with slow-growing, painless mass of the right thigh. Shortness of breath.

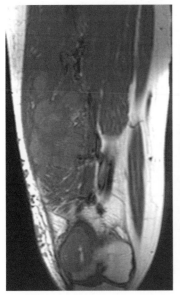

Figure 63.1

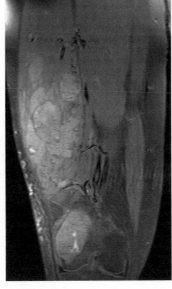

Figure 63.2

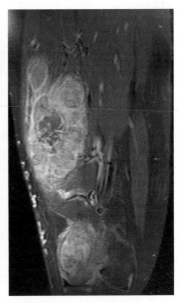

Figure 63.3

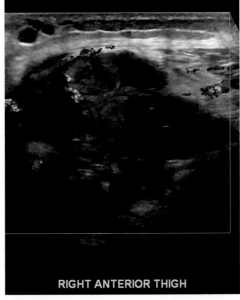

RIGHT ANTERIOR THIGH

Figure 63.4

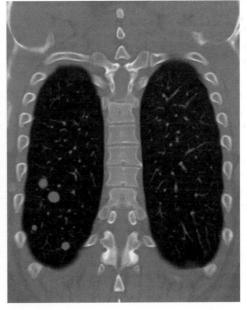

Figure 63.5

Case 63   Alveolar soft part sarcoma

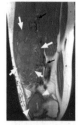 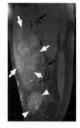 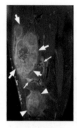 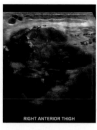 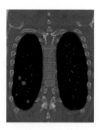

Figure 63.6   **Figure 63.7**   **Figure 63.8**   **Figure 63.9**   **Figure 63.10**

Findings

Figure 63.6 (coronal T1-weighted image) shows a heterogeneous soft tissue mass of the lateral right thigh (*white arrows all images*) with areas of increased signal intensity relative to muscle, prominent low-signal flow voids (*black arrows all images*) superior and inferior to the mass, and abnormal signal intensity in the lateral femoral condyle (*arrowheads all images*). Figures 63.7 (coronal T1-weighted FS pre-contrast image) and 63.8 (post-contrast image) show a vascular heterogeneous intramuscular lesion, prominent enhancing peripheral large feeding vessels (*small white arrows*), central necrosis, and an enhancing lateral femoral lesion. Figure 63.9 (ultrasound color Doppler) confirms the vascular nature of the mass. Figure 63.10 (coronal CT of the chest) shows round lung metastases.

Differential Diagnosis

Rhabdomyosarcoma; hemangioendothelioma or hemangiopericytoma; arteriovenous malformation; synovial sarcoma; Ewing sarcoma

Teaching Points

▶ Alveolar soft part sarcoma is a rare, malignant, slow-growing, vascular soft tissue mass of young adults, children, or adolescents (<1% of all soft tissue sarcomas).

▶ Second to fourth decades; there is a female predilection in patients <30 years and a male predilection in those >30 years.

▶ Tenderness to palpation, pulsatile sensation, or bruit may be present.

▶ In adults, it occurs more commonly in the lower extremity (thigh/buttock, calf) than in the upper extremity and retroperitoneum. In children and adolescents, head and neck location is most common.

▶ Radiographs: normal, soft tissue swelling, occasionally calcification

▶ MR/CT/US: Heterogeneous soft tissue mass isointense/hyperintense to muscle (T1), atypical regions of high T1/T2 signal (blood), multiple flow voids (large feeding vessels) at the core and periphery and marked enhancement with central necrosis. Highly vascular hypoechoic soft tissue mass (color Doppler) with low resistive index.

▶ Metastases (chest>brain, bone) occur early and are common at presentation (33%).

▶ Chest radiograph/CT if alveolar soft part sarcoma is suspected. Bone involvement is uncommon (multiple or solitary).

Management

Staging is key. Chest and intracranial imaging evaluation should be done at presentation to identify metastases. Treatment involves radical wide resection with adjuvant radiation/chemotherapy (65% 5-year survival). There is a worse prognosis for patients who are older or who have metastases at diagnosis or lesions >5 cm. Biopsy may cause extensive bleeding; embolization may be required before sampling.

Further Readings

Iwamoto Y, Morimoto N, Chuman H, Shinohara N, Sugioka Y. The role of MR imaging in the diagnosis of alveolar soft part sarcoma: a report of 10 cases. *Skeletal Radiol* 1995;24(4):257–270.

Murphey MD, Kransdorf MJ. Chapter 12: Tumors of uncertain histogenesis. In *Imaging of Soft Tissue Tumors*, 2nd ed. Philadelphia: Lippincott Williams and Wilkins, 2006:493–497.

History

▶ 34-year-old man with a 1-year history of progressive fullness of the left axilla with painless enlarging mass and decreased range of motion of the left shoulder

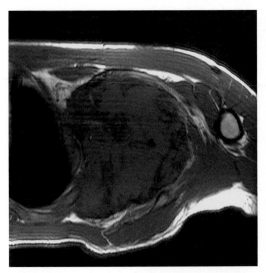

Figure 64.1

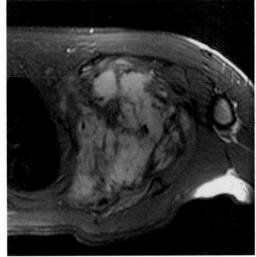

Figure 64.2

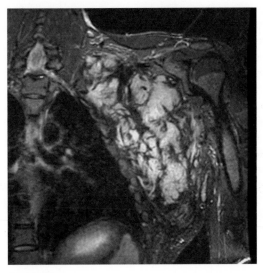

Figure 64.3

Case 64 Aggressive fibromatosis (deep fibromatosis or extra-abdominal desmoid)

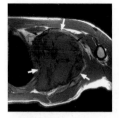 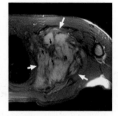 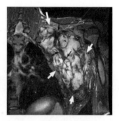

Figure 64.4   **Figure 64.5**   **Figure 64.6**

Findings

Figures 64.4 through 64.6 (axial T1-weighted, T1-weighted fat-saturated post-gadolinium, and coronal STIR weighted MR images of the left axilla) demonstrate a large heterogeneous soft tissue mass in the intermuscular region of the left axilla (*white arrows*) with low-intermediate T1-signal, nonenhancing collagenized foci peripherally and centrally that persist on all images (*black arrows*), diffuse increased signal within the mass on STIR and post-gadolinium sequences, and diffuse enhancement of remaining areas. Left shoulder radiograph (not shown) showed prominence of axillary soft tissues without mineralization, bone abnormality, or gas.

Differential Diagnosis

Malignant fibrous histiocytoma; sarcoma

Teaching Points

▶ Deep fibromatoses are benign, relatively common soft tissue lesions that affect fascia, septa, and aponeurosis between muscles. Rare cases may have synchronous lesions, and 10% are multifocal.

▶ Typically presents in young adults (puberty to 40 years old) as a slow-growing, painless soft tissue mass with a predilection for women. Symptoms may include limited range of motion or neurologic symptoms.

▶ 70% occur in the extremities, specifically shoulder, chest wall/paraspinal, thigh, head/neck, knee, buttock, hip, lower leg, and forearm, in decreasing order of frequency.

▶ Imaging appearance is often aggressive, but these lesions do not metastasize. They are associated with a high local recurrence rate (19% to 77%).

▶ Axillary lesions often surround neurovascular structures and are not amenable to resection.

▶ *Radiographs*: Soft tissue mass; rare bone involvement (scalloping or pressure erosion)

▶ *CT*: Variable attenuation, often with low-attenuation collagenized areas that do not enhance. Increased capillary network contributes to diffuse enhancement of remainder of lesion.

▶ *MR*: Low-signal-intensity areas on all sequences due to collagen and hypocellularity but may have diffuse high T2 or STIR signal if higher cellularity. Margins are smooth or infiltrative and can invade muscle with extension of fascial tail along the fascia. This "tail" helps to distinguish a desmoid lesion and is important to mention in the radiology report to allow for complete resection.

Management

Localized radiation is the preferred treatment, particularly in cases not amenable to wide resection. Lesions demonstrating progressive collagenization with low signal intensity on all pulse sequences following therapy do not require surgical management; those with increased size and persistent high signal after therapy require surgical resection if lesion is amenable. Chemotherapy has proven effective in aggressive cases. Anti-inflammatories and antiestrogens have shown success in nonresponsive lesions.

Further Readings

Ackman JB, Whiteman G, Chew FS. Aggressive fibromatosis. *AJR Am J Roentgenol* 1994;*163*:544.

Kransdorf MJ, Murphey MD. Benign fibrous and fibrohistiocytic tumors. In *Imaging of Soft Tissue Tumors*, 2nd ed. Philadelphia: Lippincott Williams and Wilkins, 2006:188–256.

Lee JC, Thomas JM, Phillips S, Fisher C, Moskovic E. Aggressive fibromatosis: MRI features with pathologic correlation. *AJR Am J Roentgenol* 2006;*186*:247–254.

History

▶ Wrist pain, fullness, and swelling

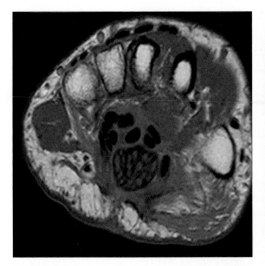

Figure 65.1

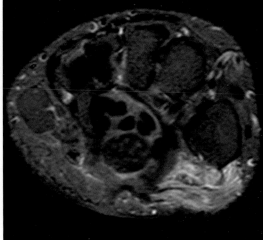

Figure 65.2

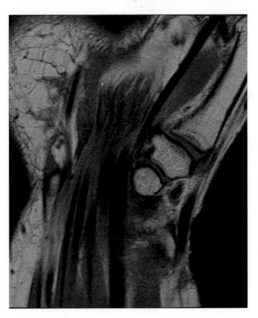

Figure 65.3

Case 65   Fibrolipomatous hamartoma of the median nerve with resultant carpal tunnel syndrome

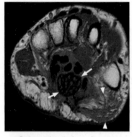

Figure 65.4

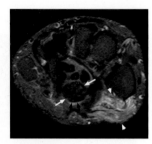

Figure 65.5

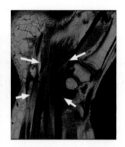

Figure 65.6

Findings

Figures 65.4 and 65.5 (axial T1-weighted and STIR MR images of the distal wrist), and 65.6 (coronal T1-weighted MR wrist): Abnormal enlargement of the median nerve (*white arrows*) with serpiginous low-signal-intensity material and alternating high/intermediate material suggesting nerve fascicles, fibrous tissue and fat. Associated volar bowing of the flexor retinaculum (*small black arrows*) is present with minimal fluid within surrounding otherwise normal appearing flexor tendons within the carpal tunnel on the STIR image. The axial images also demonstrate mild fatty atrophy (T1) and diffuse edema (STIR) within the thenar muscles (*arrowheads*).

Differential Diagnosis

Fatty infiltration; neuritis; onspecific mass; infection, inflammation; neurofibroma

Teaching Points

▶ The median nerve is the only nerve within the carpal tunnel at the radial volar aspect alongside the flexor tendons. Normally it is oval and smooth with mild increased signal intensity on all sequences in comparison to adjacent tendons.
▶ T1-weighted images are best for confirming fat-containing fusiform mass with a low-signal-intensity "spaghetti-like" appearance of nerve fascicles, interspersed fat, and fibrous tissue.
▶ Axial images demonstrate pathognomonic "coaxial cable-like" appearance of the median nerve.
▶ Denervation edema within the thenar muscles (best seen on fluid sensitive sequences) helps to confirm median nerve involvement.
▶ This is a space-occupying lesion within the carpal tunnel that can contribute to carpal tunnel syndrome or symptoms. (Other causes of carpal tunnel syndrome are listed in the differential above).
▶ The adjacent flexor tendons are usually unremarkable but may demonstrate some degree of tendinopathy due to compression by the enlarged nerve.
▶ Bowing of the low signal flexor retinaculum may be seen in carpal tunnel syndrome.

Further Readings

De Maesseneer M, Jaovisidha S, Lenchik L, Witte L, Schweizter M, Sartoris D, Resnik D. Fibrolipomatous hamartoma: MR imaging findings. *Skeletal Radiol* 1997;*26*(3):155–160.
Marom EM, Helms C. Fibrolipomatous hamartoma: pathognomonic on MR imaging. *Skeletal Radiol* 1999;*28*(5):260–264.

History

► Patient with breast cancer and left shoulder pain

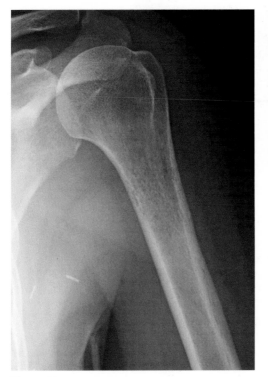

Figure 66.1

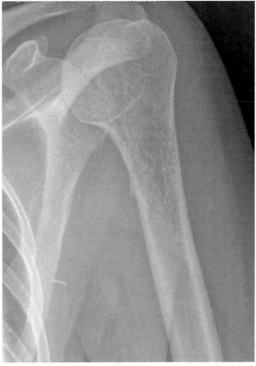

Figure 66.2

Case 66 Metastatic lesion, left humerus, with development of a pathologic fracture

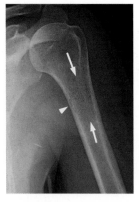

Figure 66.3

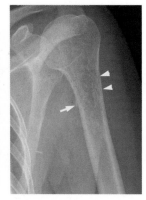

figure 66.4

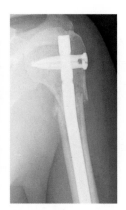

Figure 66.5

Findings

Figure 66.3 (frontal radiograph of the proximal left humerus) reveals a subtle, permeative lytic lesion in its proximal shaft (*arrows*) that demonstrates deep endosteal scalloping involving >50% of the cortex medially (*arrowhead*). The findings are most compatible with an osseous metastasis in this patient with a known history of breast cancer. Figure 66.4 (follow-up frontal radiograph of the humerus obtained 1 month later) shows worsening osteolysis at the site of the lesion with progressive lateral cortical thinning (*arrowheads*) and a small cortical fracture medially (*arrow*). Figure 66.5 (postoperative radiograph) demonstrates an intramedullary rod transfixing what is now a minimally displaced fracture.

Differential Diagnosis

Multiple myeloma; lymphoma; osteomyelitis

Teaching Points

▶ The radiographic appearance of a focal bone lesion is highly predictive of its biologic aggressiveness.
▶ A "geographic" lytic lesion demonstrates a well-defined, often sclerotic margin (the least aggressive appearance), whereas a "moth-eaten" or "permeative" pattern (as in this case) is consistent with an aggressive lesion such as neoplasm or infection.
▶ A focal bone lesion should also be assessed for radiographic features that suggest an increased risk of developing a pathologic fracture at that site. Classically, these include the following:
  – Osteolytic lesion
  – Lesion size >2.5 cm
  – Deep cortical invasion (>50% of cortical thickness)
  – Axial cortical involvement of >3 cm
  – Proximal location within the bone

Management

When one or more of these features are identified, the clinician should be notified since prophylactic stabilization will avoid the development of a displaced pathologic fracture and its associated morbidity.

Further Readings

Van der linder YM et al. Comparative analysis of risk factors for pathological fracture with femoral metastases: results based on a randomized trial of chemotherapy. *J Bone Joint Surg Br* 2004;86:566–573.

History

▶ Back pain

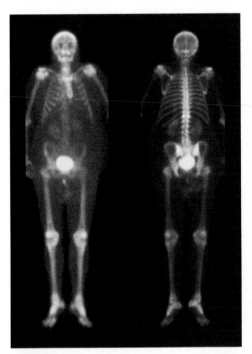

Figure 67.1

Figure 67.2

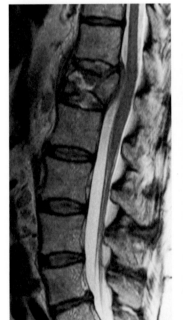

Figure 67.3

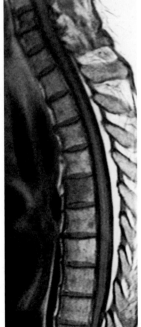

Figure 67.4

Case 67 Pathologic burst fracture (lymphoma) with additional vertebral metastases not demonstrated on the whole-body bone scan

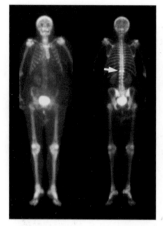 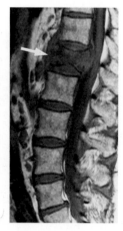 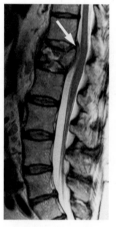 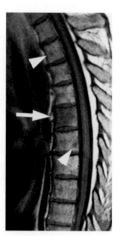

Figure 67.5   **Figure 67.6**   **Figure 67.7**   **Figure 67.8**

Findings

Anterior and posterior views from a whole-body radionuclide bone scan (Fig. 67.5) demonstrate abnormal uptake in the T12 vertebra (*arrow*), without abnormal uptake elsewhere in the spine. Sagittal T1-weighted (Fig. 67.6) and T2-weighted images (Fig. 67.7) display a pathologic burst fracture of the T12 vertebra (*arrow* in Fig. 67.6) with compression of the distal cord due to retropulsed tissue, better demonstrated on the T2-weighted image (*arrow* in Fig. 67.7). In Figure 67.8, another large metastatic focus is present in a midthoracic vertebra (*arrow*) and smaller lesions are also seen at other levels (*arrowheads*).

Differential Diagnosis

Metastatic tumor; multiple myeloma

Teaching Points

- ▶ Radionuclide bone imaging allows for rapid assessment of the entire skeleton for areas of abnormal bone turnover (tumor, fracture, infection, etc.).
- ▶ Although highly sensitive in this regard, scintigraphy has been shown to be less sensitive than MR imaging for demonstrating neoplastic involvement of the spine, which may have significant clinical implications for directing further therapy.
- ▶ Whole-body MR imaging is now available in some centers.

Management

The discovery of osseous metastases may change the initial treatment decisions for what was presumed to be a localized tumor. It may also lead to additional radiation therapy, chemotherapy, or even surgery (for an impending fracture or cord compression).

Further Readings

Ghanem N, Altehoefer C, Hogerle S, Schafer O, Winterer J, Moser E, Langer M. Comparative diagnostic value and therapeutic relevance of magnetic resonance imaging and bone marrow scintigraphy in patients with metastatic solid tumors of the axial skeleton. *Eur J Radiol* 2002;43:256–261.

Schmidt GP, Schoenberg SO, Schmid R, et al. Screening for bone metastases: whole-body MRI using a 320-channel system versus dual-modality PET-CT. *Eur Radiol* 2007;17:939–949.

Case 68

History

▶ 15-year-old with elbow pain and swelling

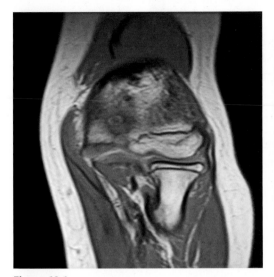

Figure 68.1

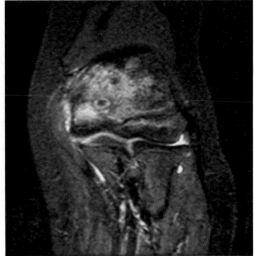

Figure 68.2

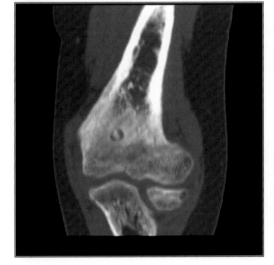

Figure 68.3

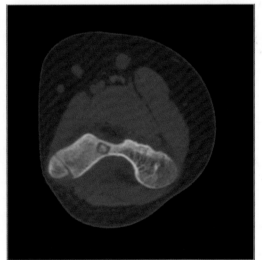

Figure 68.4

Case 68   Osteoid osteoma

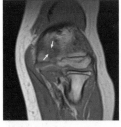

Figure 68.5

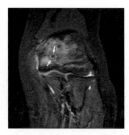

Figure 68.6

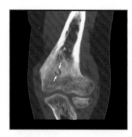

Figure 68.7

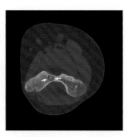

Figure 68.8

Findings

Figures 68.5 (coronal T1-weighted image) and 68.6 (coronal STIR image) of the left elbow show low T1/high STIR marrow edema of the distal humeral metaphysis surrounding a round intraosseous lesion with a central nidus (*white arrows*) (isointense to muscle on T1). Figures 68.7 (coronal CT) and 68.8 (axial CT) best demonstrate an intraosseous, well-defined, round, lucent distal humeral metaphyseal lesion with a central mineralized nidus (*white arrows*).

Differential Diagnosis

Foreign body reaction; Brodie's abscess; bone island or osteoblastoma; stress fracture (marrow edema)

Teaching Points

▸ Osteoid osteoma is a benign, typically cortical (80%) bone lesion with a characteristic central hypervascular nidus (10% of all primary bone tumors). Intramedullary or intra-articular (hip) variants occur.
▸ Location: Metaphysis (femur/tibia) (65%) > phalanges (21%) > spine (9%) > elbow
▸ Presentation: 10- to 30-year-old patient with severe night pain relieved by aspirin with or without swelling, point tenderness, or limp (children)
▸ Scoliosis (curvature toward lesion) may occur if located within the spine.
▸ *Radiographs*: Focal cortical thickening or radiolucent lesion with a central mineralized nidus, surrounding sclerosis and/or periosteal reaction
▸ *CT*: Better visualization/delineation of nidus. "Vascular groove" sign: enlarged arterioles suggest osteoid osteoma.
▸ *MR*: Diffuse marrow edema surrounding the lesion. Joint effusion or synovitis may be present with intra-articular lesions. Nidus is often isointense to muscle on T1-weighted image.
▸ *Bone scan*: "Double density" sign: Increased activity at nidus with less significant peripheral activity
▸ *US*: Cortical irregularity, hypoechoic synovitis, and pain with transducer pressure
▸ Limb overgrowth may occur if lesion is located near growth plate in children.

Management

Conservative treatment with NSAIDs with potential regression; CT-guided radioablation of the nidus; or ultimately surgical resection. Incomplete removal can lead to recurrence. Previous therapy included alcohol ablation.

Further Readings

Ebrahim FS, Jacobson JA, Lin J, Housner JA, Hayes CW, Resnick D. Intraarticular osteoid osteoma—sonographic findings in three patients with radiographic, CT and MR correlation. *AJR Am J Roentgenol* 2001;*177*:1391–1395.
Liu PT, Kujak JL, Roberts CC, de Chadarevian JP. The vascular groove sign: A new CT findings associated with osteoid osteomas. *AJR Am J Roentgenol* 2011;*196*(1):168–173.
Moser RP, Kransdorf KJ, Brower AC, et al. Osteoid osteoma of the elbow: a review of 6 cases. *Skeletal Radiol* 1990;*19*:181–186.

History

▸ 28-year-old man with tender palpable mass of the left upper arm

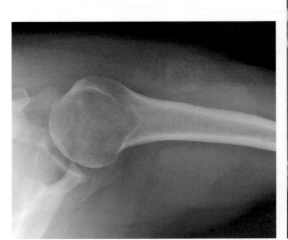

Figure 69.1

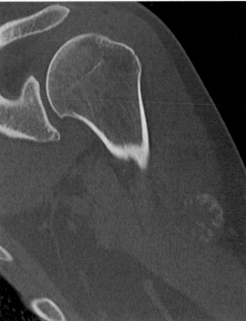

Figure 69.2

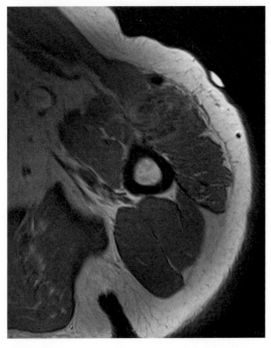

Figure 69.3

Case 69 Myositis ossificans

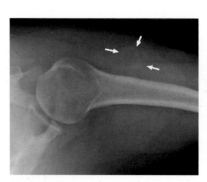

Figure 69.4

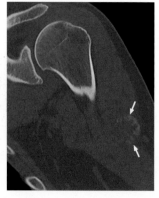

Figure 69.5

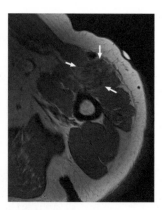

Figure 69.6

Findings

Figure 69.4 (Shoulder radiograph axillary view) demonstrates focal area of soft tissue mineralization with predominantly peripheral ossification (zonal phenomenon) (*white arrows*) within the lateral soft tissues, adjacent to but not contiguous with the proximal humerus. Figure 69.5 (coronal CT) better delineates the peripheral ossification (*white arrows*) within the deltoid muscle without other findings. Figure 69.6 (axial T1-weighted MR) demonstrates an intramuscular heterogeneous lesion with faint peripheral low signal intensity (*white arrows*). No other findings.

Differential Diagnosis

Soft tissue sarcoma; parosteal osteosarcoma (but no central ossification and not attached to bone); chondroma; healing soft tissue infection

Teaching Points

▶ Myositis ossificans is a benign soft tissue lesion that can be idiopathic or secondary to trauma.

▶ It is characterized by a zonal phenomenon of peripheral ossification best seen on CT or radiographs. It may be entirely within soft tissues or may have a small attachment to cortical bone. Peripheral zonal mineralization helps to distinguish it from the central mineralization of parosteal osteosarcoma.

▶ MR can be useful but confusing. Early-stage myositis ossificans appears as a soft tissue mass often isointense to muscle or as a complex hematoma with hemosiderin with adjacent soft tissue edema. After 8 weeks it begins to mineralize peripherally, eventually demonstrating a low-signal-intensity peripheral rim on MR. In acute and nonchronic phases, the peripheral rim demonstrates enhancement, given its vascular nature; however, mature myositis ossificans lesions do not typically enhance.

▶ Extensive soft tissue edema surrounding the lesion is characteristic in early phases; this helps differentiate it from soft tissue sarcoma, which typically does not have surrounding soft tissue edema.

▶ In lesions immediately adjacent to bone, a cleft between the calcified mass and the cortex will form over time; this helps to confirm the benign nature.

Management

No treatment is needed unless there is secondary nerve or vascular structure compression or cosmetic deformity.

Further Readings

Kransdorf MJ, Meis JM, Jelinek JS. Myositis ossificans: MR appearance with radiologic–pathologic correlation. *AJR Am J Roentgenol* 1991;*157*:1243–1248.

Mulcahy H, Chew FS. MRI of non-tumorous skeletal muscle disease: a case-based review. *AJR Am J Roentgenol* 2011;*196*(6):S77–S85.

History

▶ Right thigh pain and swelling status post gunshot wound with decreasing hematocrit

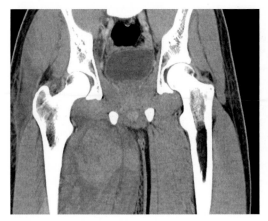

Figure 70.1

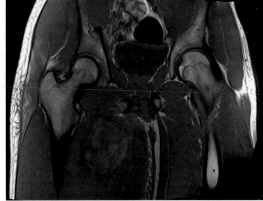

Figure 70.2

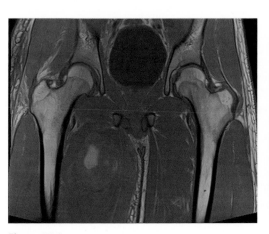

Figure 70.3

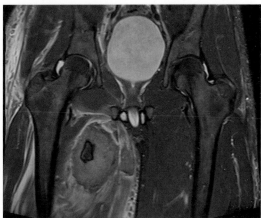

Figure 70.4

Case 70   Hematoma

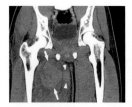
Figure 70.5

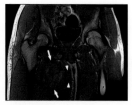
Figure 70.6

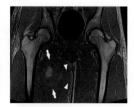
Figure 70.7

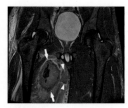
Figure 70.8

Findings

Figures 70.5 (coronal CT) and 70.6 (coronal T1) show a well-defined fluid collection (*arrows*) with a smaller adjacent collection (*arrowheads)* within the medial compartment of the right thigh demonstrating increased density on CT and increased heterogeneous T1 signal intensity. Follow up coronal MR images obtained five days later (Figures 70.7 – T1; 70.8 – STIR) reveal heterogeneous signal intensity within the collection as well as a central focus of high signal intensity on T1 that shows low signal intensity on the STIR image compatible with subacute hemorrhage (*black arrows*).

Differential Diagnosis

Hemorrhage within tumor

Teaching Points

► Hematoma is a discrete collection of blood confined to a restricted location. CT, MR and ultrasound are useful for diagnosis. US may be utilized for sampling or drainage if required.
► MR appearance varies depending upon time frame of imaging:
  ▪ Hyperacute (<24 hours)—isointense/slightly higher than muscle (T1); hyperintense (T2)
  ▪ Acute (1 to 3 days)—isointense/slightly higher than muscle (T1); dark (T2)
  ▪ Early subacute (>3 days)—bright (T1); dark (T2)
  ▪ Late subacute (>7 days)—bright (T1); bright (T2)
  ▪ Chronic (>14 days)—dark (T1); dark (T2)
► Initial imaging in this case demonstrated findings of an acute hematoma from transaction of a femoral vessel and then features of subacute hemorrhage on the follow up images.
► In older patients or in those without a history of trauma or bleeding history, exclude underlying tumor that has led to hemorrhage.

Management

Evaluation of vessel integrity with potential embolization for active extravasation in cases of progressing hematoma and falling hematocrit. Follow-up imaging to resolution is recommended to exclude an underlying tumor in older patients or patients without an underlying history of trauma or bleeding disorders. Image guided drainage or biopsy may be required if the hematoma is compressing adjacent structures or if it does not resolve.

Further Readings

Bush CH. The magnetic resonance imaging of musculoskeletal hemorrhage. *Skeletal Radiol* 2000;*29*(1):1–9.
Gilbert BC, Bui-Mansfield L, Dejong S. MRI of a Morel-Lavalée lesion. *AJR Am J Roentgenol* 2004;*184*(5):1347–1348.
Lee YS, Kwon ST, Kim JO. Serial MR imaging of intramuscular hematoma: Experimental study in a rat model with the pathologic correlation. *Korean J Radiol* 2011;*12*(1):66–77.

Part III   Infection

History

▶ 3-year-old with a limp

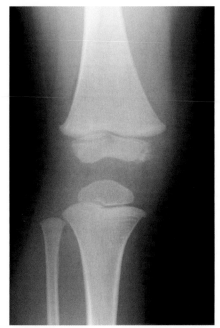

Figure 71.1

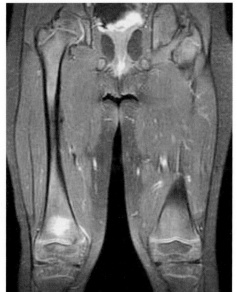

Figure 71.2

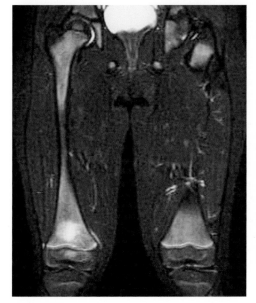

Figure 71.3

Figure 71.4

Case 71 Acute osteomyelitis

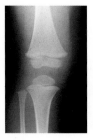

Figure 71.5

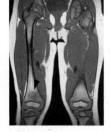

Figure 71.6

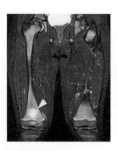

Figure 71.7

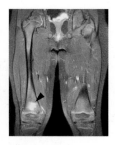

Figure 71.8

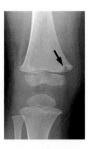

Figure 71.9

Findings

Figure 71.5 (initial PA radiograph) is normal. Coronal T1-weighted image (Fig. 71.6), STIR image (Fig. 71.7), and contrast-enhanced fat-saturated T1-weighted image (Fig. 71.8) reveal a focus of abnormal signal intensity and enhancement in the distal femoral metaphysis (*arrowheads*), suspicious for osteomyelitis (proven by a subsequent needle biopsy: *Serratia marcescens*). Figure 71.9 (radiograph of the knee obtained 3 weeks later) demonstrates the interval development of a metaphyseal lucency at the site of infection.

Differential Diagnosis

Intramedullary tumor

Teaching Points

▶ Acute osteomyelitis in children usually occurs via hematogenous spread; the most common offending organism is *Staphylococcus aureus*.
▶ The metaphysis of a long bone is the site most commonly affected, probably related to the tortuous, slowly flowing vessels in that region.
▶ Bacteria may spread to the epiphysis via transphyseal vessels, but this is less commonly seen after these vessels close between the ages of 12 and 18 months.
▶ Intramedullary or subperiosteal abscesses may develop, and infection of an adjacent joint may occur.
▶ Given the potentially aggressive imaging appearance of osteomyelitis, percutaneous biopsy may be necessary to exclude malignancy in some cases.

Management

Intravenous antibiotics. Surgical intervention may be required, especially in the case of a septic joint or loculated abscess.

Further Readings

Blickman JG, van Die CE, de Rooy JWJ. Current imaging concepts in pediatric osteomyelitis. *Eur Radiol* 2004;*14*:L55–L64.
Karmazyn B. Imaging approach to acute hematogenous osteomyelitis in children: an update. *Semin Ultrasound CT MRI* 2010;*31*:100–106.

History

▸ 38-year-old man with persistent low back pain and recurrent visits to the emergency department

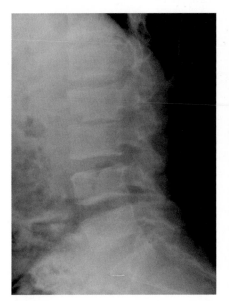

Figure 72.1

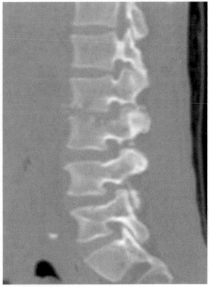

Figure 72.2

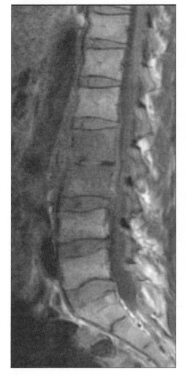

Figure 72.3

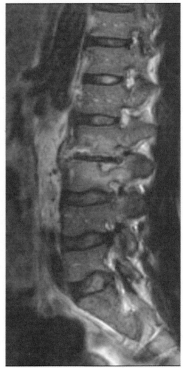

Figure 72.4

Case 72 Spondylodiskitis, bacterial L2-L3 (*Staphylococcus*)

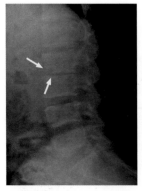 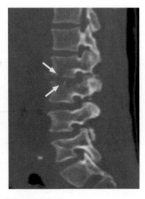 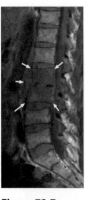 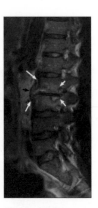

Figure 72.5   **Figure 72.6**   **Figure 72.7**   **Figure 72.8**

Findings

Figures 72.5 (lateral lumbar spine radiograph) and 72.6 (sagittal CT) show irregularity and cortical destruction of the endplates bordering the L2–L3 disk space (*white arrows*) with associated narrowing of the disk space itself. Figures 72.7 (sagittal T1-weighted MR image) and 72.8 (sagittal T2-weighted MR image) show abnormal signal intensity within the L2–3 disk space and adjacent vertebral bodies (low on T1 and increased on T2) with focal anterior soft tissue prominence (*black arrow*).

Differential Diagnosis

Typically pathognomonic of spondylodiskitis. (Amyloid, particularly hemodialysis spondyloarthropathy, or gout could be included in the differential, but a lack of 10-year history of hemodialysis and lack of overhanging margins or sclerotic rims about potential erosions make these diagnoses very unlikely.)

Teaching Points

▶ Spinal infection begins in the sub-endplate regions of the vertebral body, extending to the adjacent vertebral endplate and disk. Irregularity and cortical destruction of the adjacent endplates with decreased height of the corresponding disk are pathognomonic, with characteristic MR signal changes involving disk and marrow as noted in this case. There is sclerosis of the destroyed endplates in the chronic phase.
▶ Hematogenous spread is most common. If it involves only the disk (particularly in skeletally immature patients), it is called diskitis and may be self-limited.
▶ Patient may have associated paravertebral or epidural mass or displaced psoas shadow.
▶ Genitourinary infections can be frequent cause of spine infections.
▶ TB infections in comparison are characterized by subligamentous spread (which may involve many levels), preservation of the disk space, lack of a sclerotic response, and thoracolumbar predominance.
▶ Chronic recurrent osteomyelitis CROM lesions may mimic spondylodiskitis, but they do not typically cross the disk space, which helps distinguish between the two entities.
▶ Contrast-enhanced MR helps to identify an abscess within the disk or epidural space.

Management

IV antibiotics. Biopsy (bone or disk) if needed to determine specific organism and further tailor treatment. Surgical intervention if no improvement or severe.

Further Readings

Ledermann H et al. MR imaging findings in spinal infections: Rules or myths. *Radiographics* 2003;228:506–514.
Stabler A, Reiser MF. Imaging of spinal infection. *Radiol Clin North Am* 2001;39:115–135.

History

▶ 42-year-old man with right hip pain and limp

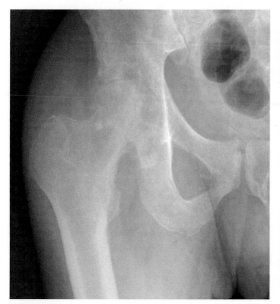

Figure 73.1

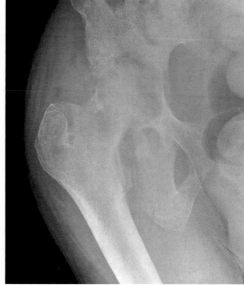

Figure 73.2

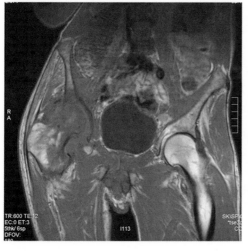

Figure 73.3

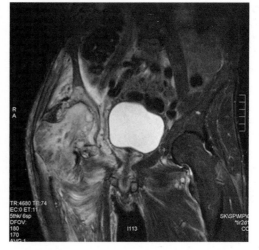

Figure 73.4

Case 73 Septic arthritis with osteomyelitis

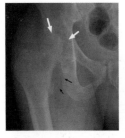

Figure 73.5

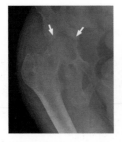

Figure 73.6

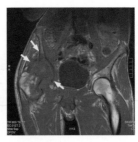

Figure 73.7

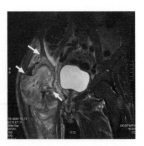

Figure 73.8

Findings

Figure 73.5 (initial AP radiograph) demonstrates decreased bone density of the right femoral head and adjacent acetabulum with loss of femoral head cortical visualization and narrowing of the joint space (*white arrows*). Mild bowing of the inferomedial fat plane between the joint space and adjacent muscle (*black arrows*) suggests joint fluid. Figure 73.6 (AP radiograph2 months later) demonstrates rapid loss of bone density with disruption of the joint space and bone destruction on both sides of the joint. Figure 73.7 (T1-weighted coronal MR image) displays abnormal low signal intensity throughout the entire proximal femur, adjacent right acetabulum and ischium/superior pubic ramus junction, with loss of right hip joint space and loss of visualization of the cortical margins (*white arrows*) Figure 73.8 (STIR coronal MR image) demonstrates abnormal high signal intensity throughout the right femur and acetabulum, high-signal fluid within the narrowed joint space, multifocal high-signal collections in bone, and diffuse edema within the adjacent muscles.

Differential Diagnosis

Radiography: infection (septic arthritis), malignancy, transient osteoporosis. MR imaging: infection (septic arthritis + osteomyelitis), malignancy.

Teaching Points

▶ Radiographic evidence of rapid loss of bone density on both sides of a joint, initial joint space widening followed by joint space narrowing and associated displacement of fat pads to suggest joint fluid are characteristic of septic arthritis.

▶ As disease advances, focal cortical destruction of bone can occur with progression of disease leading to advanced osteomyelitis with possible sinus tracts or intraosseous foci of infection, as in this case.

▶ While transient osteoporosis can present with severe hip pain and diffuse bone density loss of the proximal femur, it can be differentiated from septic arthritis by its lack of the following features: involvement of the adjacent acetabulum, cortical destruction, focal intraosseous lesions on MRI, and muscle involvement.

▶ *Staphylococcus aureus* is the most common etiologic agent.

▶ Malignancy can have diffuse marrow involvement, but it rarely crosses joints, with the exceptions of giant cell tumor, chordoma of the spine, or rarely leukemia and lymphoma.

Management

Image-guided aspiration of the hip joint followed by culture-guided intravenous antibiotic therapy. Bone biopsy of affected areas is usually not required but may be utilized if cultures are negative.

Further Readings

Karchevsky M, Schweitzer M, Morrison W, Parellada J. MR findings of septic arthritis and associated osteomyelitis in adults. *AJR Am J Roentgenol* 2004;*182*:119–122.

Resnick D. *Bone and Joint Imaging*. Philadelphia: WB Saunders Co., 1989:744–749.

History

► Right buttock, back, and pelvic pain in patient with history of MRSA

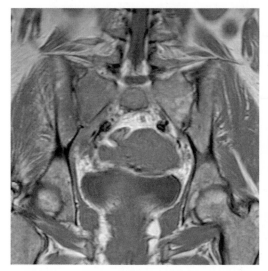

Figure 74.1

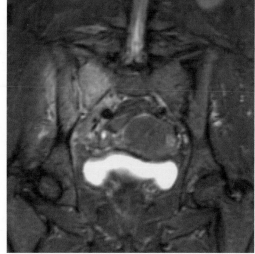

Figure 74.2

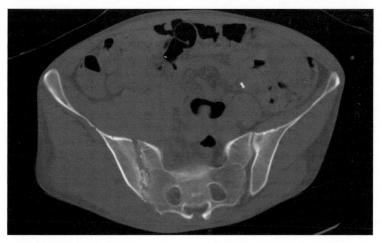

Figure 74.3

Case 74   Unilateral septic sacroiliitis

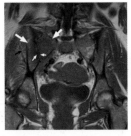

Figure 74.4

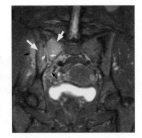

Figure 74.5

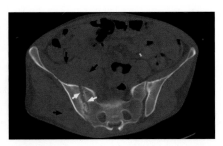

Figure 74.6

Findings

Figures 74.4 and 74.5 (coronal T1-weighted and STIR MR images) demonstrate abnormal low-T1-signal-intensity/high-STIR-signal-intensity bone marrow edema on both sides of the right sacroiliac joint (*white arrows*) with widening of the mid-inferior right sacroiliac joint and associated intra-articular fluid (*small white arrows*). Adjacent gluteal and iliopsoas muscle edema and swelling is present (*black arrows*). Figure 74.6 (axial CT) better depicts the cortical destruction and widening of the right sacroiliac joint (*white arrows*) with further enlargement of the involved iliopsoas muscle and posterior gluteal muscles.

Differential Diagnosis

Unilateral seronegative sacroiliitis; (rare cases of lymphoma or Ewing sarcoma)

Teaching Points

▶ Pyogenic sacroiliitis represents 1% to 2% of all infections, most commonly *Staphylococcus aureus*, and is unilateral. (The differential diagnosis for bilateral sacroiliitis includes ankylosing spondylitis, enteropathic spondylitis, and psoriasis.)

▶ MR findings: Bone marrow signal abnormality on both the sacral and iliac sides of the joint, typically involving the mid-inferior portion of the joint, irregular widening of the joint space, and intra-articular fluid should suggest infection in the appropriate clinical setting.

▶ Associated intramuscular abscesses or myositis are common and can be better appreciated using post-contrast MR or CT imaging. Joint fluid typically does not enhance. Presence of gas may suggest infection; however, intra-articular gas can also be seen with previous articular trauma or as vacuum phenomenon in osteoarthritis.

▶ The erosions seen in seronegative spondyloarthropathies with associated marrow edema can mimic infectious sacroiliitis, but the presence of joint fluid and intramuscular abscesses should point to an infectious etiology.

▶ Radiographs may demonstrate cortical irregularity or destruction of the unilateral sacroiliac joint with or without lytic or sclerotic ossific changes on both sides of the sacroiliac joint; however, they are often insensitive due to overlying bowel gas and stool.

▶ Rare instances of lymphoma or Ewing sarcoma involving the iliac bone adjacent to the SI joint may mimic unilateral septic sacroiliitis however the presence of soft tissue mass and normal joint space help exclude these processes.

Management

CT and MRI help determine the extent of bone, joint, and muscle involvement as well as direct image-guided aspiration of fluid or biopsy of tissue for diagnosis and tailoring of antibiotic treatment. Advanced imaging can also direct drain placement for relief of symptoms. High dose oral and IV antibiotics are mainstay of treatment. Surgery is performed if there is a need for open biopsy and abscess drainage.

Further Readings

Long S, Yablon C, Eisenberg R. Bone marrow signal alteration in the spine and sacrum. *AJR Am J Roentgenol* 2011;*195*:W175–W200.

Murphey MD, Wetzel LH, Bramble JM, et al. Sacroiliitis: MR imaging findings. *Radiology* 1991;*180*:239–244.

Case 75

History

- Immunosuppressed 36-year-old man with fevers of unknown origin and bilateral calf pain and swelling

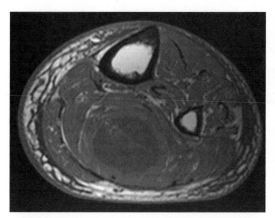

Figure 75.1

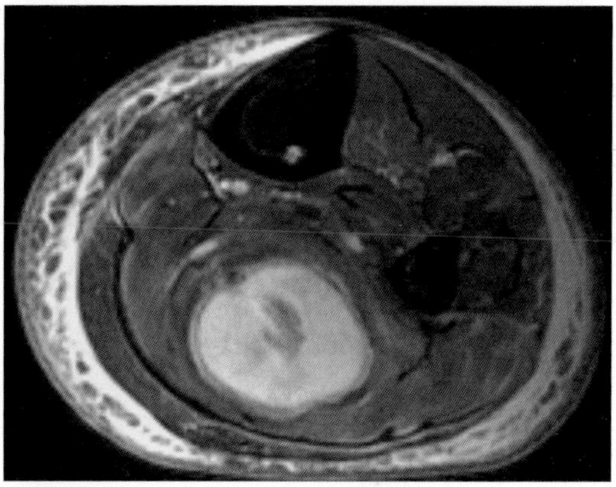

Figure 75.2

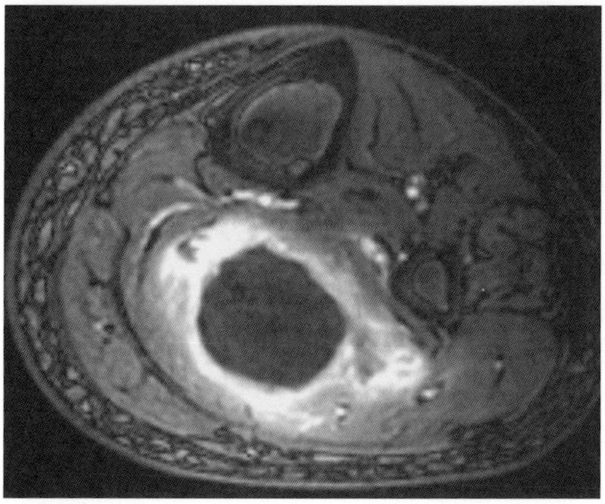

Figure 75.3

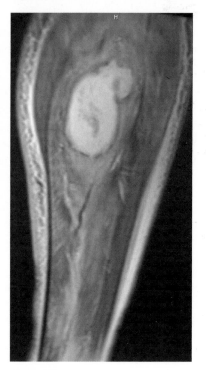

Figure 75.4

Case 75 Intramuscular soft tissue abscess/pyomyositis— *Staphylococcus aureus*

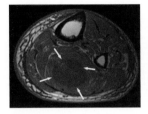

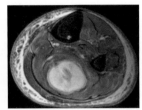

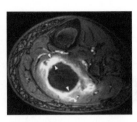

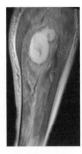

Figure 75.5   **Figure 75.6**   **Figure 75.7**   **Figure 75.8**

Findings

Figure 75.5 (axial T1-weighted MR image of the calf) depicts a focal intramuscular fluid collection with signal intensity lower than adjacent muscle (*white arrows*). Diffuse subcutaneous edema is present. Figure 75.6 (axial T2-weighted fat-saturated MR image) demonstrates diffuse bright signal intensity throughout the collection (*white arrows*) with a thick rim and edema within the adjacent muscles and overlying subcutaneous fat. Axial T1-weighted post-gadolinium MR image (Fig. 75.7) demonstrates a thick peripheral rim of enhancement (*arrowheads*) surrounding the low-T1-signal-intensity fluid collection, with the sagittal STIR MR image (Fig. 75.8) best demonstrating diffuse posterior compartment muscle edema and diffuse subcutaneous edema surrounding the T2-bright heterogeneous intramuscular collection.

Differential Diagnosis

Hematoma; sarcoma; myxoid lesion

Teaching Points

▶ Abscesses are localized collections of pus within a confined space that become walled off by vascularized connective tissues over time. Pyomyositis refers to a primary bacterial infection involving skeletal muscle that is often seen in immunocompromised patients. Gas (best seen on CT or gradient echo MR), fluid–fluid levels, and diffuse inflammation, swelling of fascial planes, and subcutaneous fat stranding are common findings.

▶ Causes include trauma, contamination from a septic focus, or hematogenous dissemination.

▶ Radiographs may demonstrate soft tissue prominence or gas. CT shows an enlarged muscle, fluid attenuation mass, with or without gas, with an enhancing thick peripheral capsule. MR provides better visualization than CT, helping to distinguish between cellulitis and soft tissue abscess(es).demonstrating a well-demarcated collection of increased T2 signal intensity and decreased T1 signal intensity with a thick rim of variable signal intensity (typically higher signal intensity than muscle on T1 that enhances). MR helps to distinguish from hematoma (bright as fat on T1 in the acute setting) and phlegmon (no focal fluid collection but only inflammatory edema pattern). Signal void within the collection suggests a foreign body.

▶ Ultrasound shows variable echogenicity (anechoic if liquefied to variable if foreign material or gas) with hyperemia within the thick wall on Doppler ultrasound; however, it may be indistinguishable from hematoma.

Management

Ultrasound is useful for diagnosis as well as percutaneous aspiration/drainage. Treatment includes intravenous antibiotics based on culture and sensitivity of fluid obtained.

Further Readings

Kransdorf MJ, Murphey MD. Masses that may mimic soft tissue tumors. In *Imaging of Soft Tissue Tumors*, 2nd ed. Philadelphia: Lippincott Williams and Wilkins, 2006:511–572.

Yu CW et al. Bacterial pyomyositis: MRI and clinical correlation. *Magnetic Resonance Imaging* 2004;22(9):1233–1241.

History

▶ Cellulitis

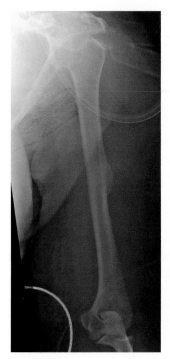
Figure 76.1

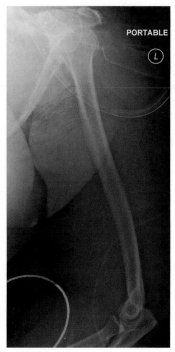
Figure 76.2

Case 76   Necrotizing fasciitis

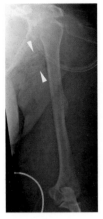

Figure 76.3

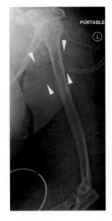

Figure 76.4

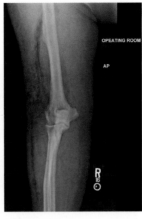

Figure 76.5

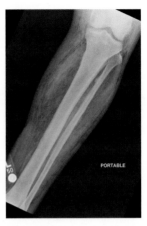

Figure 76.6

Findings

AP radiographs of the left humerus (Fig. 76.3, external rotation; Fig. 76.4, internal rotation) demonstrate prominent gas dissecting within the soft tissues of the upper arm and axilla (*arrowheads*). AP radiographs of the right elbow (Fig. 76.5) and the left lower leg (Fig. 76.6) reveal even more prominent soft tissue gas in these extremities, consistent with widespread necrotizing fasciitis. Despite extensive débridement, the patient died within 48 hours of these films.

Differential Diagnosis

Other types of gas-forming infections

Teaching Points

▶ Necrotizing fasciitis is a virulent soft tissue infection produced by a variety of bacteria that are introduced by direct implantation through the skin or via hematogenous spread. While it most commonly afflicts diabetic and immunocompromised patients, it can also occur in young, healthy individuals.

▶ Initial clinical signs and symptoms may be subtle, but early diagnosis is essential since the rapid development of systemic toxicity is common and the disease is often fatal unless treated early in its course.

▶ Although most cases do not involve gas-forming organisms, the radiographic finding of soft tissue gas is considered to be diagnostic in a patient with a suspicious clinical presentation. CT scanning is even more sensitive in this regard.

▶ MR imaging has been used to differentiate necrotizing fasciitis from pyomyositis and other noninfectious types of fasciitis. (See references for more detail.)

Management

Antibiotic therapy and early surgical intervention consisting of débridement and/or amputation of the affected areas.

Further Readings

Green RJ, Dafoe DC, Raffin TA. Necrotizing fasciitis. *Chest* 1996;*110*:219–229.

Kim K-T, Kim YJ, Lee JW, et al. Can necrotizing infectious fasciitis be differentiated from nonnecrotizing infectious fasciitis with MR imaging? *Radiology* 2011;*259*:816–824.

Seok JH, Jee W-H, Chun K-A, et al. Necrotizing fasciitis versus pyomyositis: discrimination with using MR imaging. *Korean J Radiol* 2009;*10*:121–128.

History

▶ Child with extremity pain

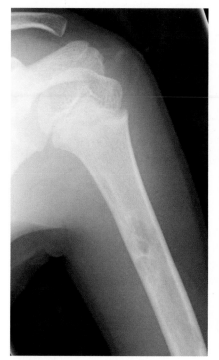

Figure 77.1

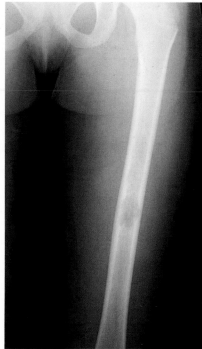

Figure 77.2

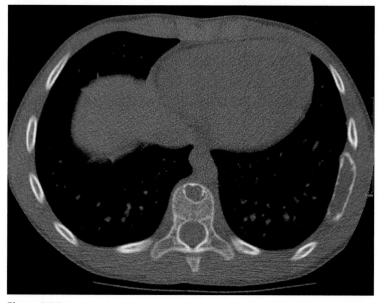

Figure 77.3

Case 77 Cystic angiomatosis

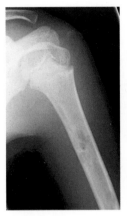

Figure 77.4

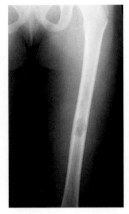

Figure 77.5

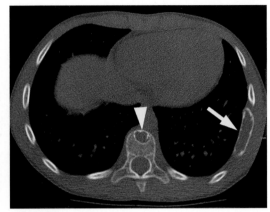

Figure 77.6

Findings

Figure 77.4 (AP image of the proximal humerus) demonstrates several relatively well-defined, multilobular lytic lesions within the humeral shaft, some of which demonstrate sclerotic margins. Figure 77.5 (AP view of the left femur) shows a similar mid-shaft lesion. Figure 77.6 (axial CT scan through the chest without intravenous contrast) reveals a well-circumscribed lytic lesion within a lower thoracic vertebral body (*arrowhead*) as well as an expansile lytic lesion in an adjacent rib (*arrow*).

Differential Diagnosis

Lymphangiomatosis; Langerhans cell histiocytosis; enchondromatosis; polyostotic fibrous dysplasia

Teaching Points

▶ Cystic angiomatosis is an idiopathic disorder in which angiomatous masses are found in bone, and often viscera as well (60% to 70% of patients).

▶ Patients typically present before the age of 30.

▶ Radiographs reveal well-circumscribed, lytic lesions, sometimes described as having a "honeycomb" or "hole within a hole" appearance, often with sclerotic margins.

▶ Definitive diagnosis may be elusive via needle biopsy given the relative paucity of solid tissue within these lesions.

Management

Laser therapy; surgical resection (possibly with preoperative embolization)

Further Readings

Murphey MD, Fairbairn KJ, Parman LM, Baxter KG, Parsa MB, Smith WS. Musculoskeletal angiomatous lesions: radiologic-pathologic correlation. *Radiographics*1995;*15*:893–917.

Part IV   Trauma and Other

History

▶ Status post wrist injury

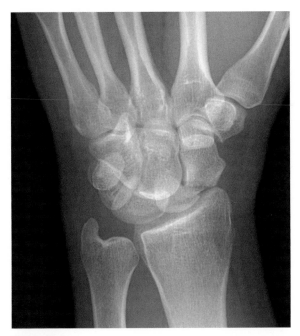

Figure 78.1

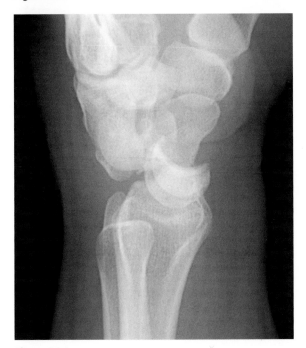

Figure 78.2

Case 78 Transscaphoid perilunate fracture-dislocation

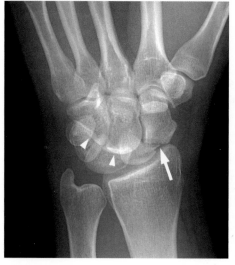

Figure 78.3

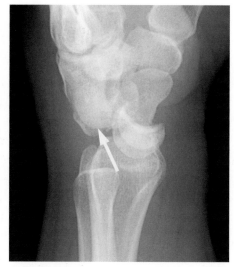

Figure 78.4

Findings

Figure 78.3 (PA radiograph of the wrist) demonstrates abnormal overlap of the proximal and distal carpal rows (*arrowheads*) and a displaced midscaphoid fracture (*arrow*). Figure 78.4 (lateral view) shows dorsal dislocation of the midcarpal row (*arrow*).

Differential Diagnosis

None

Teaching Points

▶ Ligamentous injuries of the wrist occur along a spectrum from tearing of the scapholunate ligament alone to disruption of nearly all of the ligaments surrounding the lunate, resulting in a lunate dislocation.

▶ Injuries begin along the radial aspect of the wrist with either disruption of the scapholunate ligament or a fracture of the scaphoid itself.

▶ With more severe trauma, the capitolunate joint is disrupted, allowing for dorsal dislocation of the distal carpal row (perilunate dislocation), which is evident on a lateral radiograph that demonstrates dorsal displacement of the capitate, leaving an "empty" lunate, as in this case.

▶ The diagnosis may be suspected on an AP radiograph when there is abnormal overlap of the proximal and distal carpal rows ("carpal crowding").

▶ CT may be needed for preoperative planning.

Management

Closed reduction may be attempted, but operative repair is often needed. K-wire fixation is typically utilized after either open or closed procedures.

Further Readings

Forli A, Courvoisier A, Winsey S, Cocella D, Moutet F. Perilunate dislocations and transscaphoid perilunate fracture-dislocations: a retrospective study with minimum ten-year follow-up. *J Hand Surg Am* 2010;*35*:62–68.

Kaewlai R, Avery LL, Asrani AV, Abujudeh HH, Sacknoff R, Novelline RA. Multidetector CT of carpal injuries: anatomy, fractures, and fracture-dislocations. *Radiographics*. 2008;*28*:1771–1784.

History

► Forearm and wrist pain and deformity after struck by baseball bat

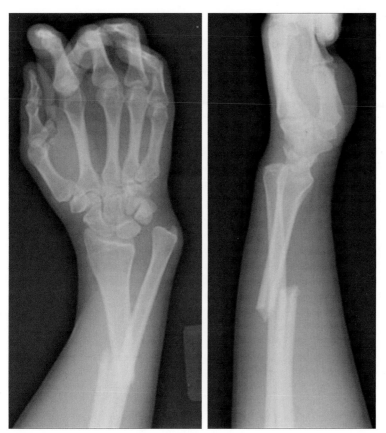

Figure 79.1

Case 79 Galeazzi fracture

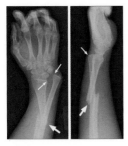

Figure 79.2

Findings

Figure 79.2 (AP and lateral wrist radiographs): Fracture of radial shaft (between middle and distal thirds) (*white arrows*) and dorsal dislocation and widening of the distal radioulnar joint (DRUJ) (*small white arrows*).

Differential Diagnosis

None

Teaching Points

▶ Galeazzi fracture-dislocation: Fracture of radial shaft (between middle and distal thirds) and associated subluxation or dislocation of DRUJ, typically in dorsal direction. Distal ulnar carpal dislocation.

▶ Fracture is almost always located just above the proximal border of the pronator quadratus on the radius.

▶ Mechanism: Typically from a fall that causes an axial load to be placed on a hyperpronated forearm (FOOSH) or direct blow.

▶ Galeazzi fractures account for 3% to 7% of all forearm fractures.

▶ Radiographic signs of DRUJ injury
  1. Ulnar styloid fracture
  2. Widening of joint on AP view
  3. Dorsal displacement on lateral view
  4. Radial shortening (~5 mm)

▶ Ulnar plus variance (radial shortening) of 10 mm or more implies complete disruption of the interosseous membrane and, therefore, complete instability of the DRUJ following reduction.

▶ CT or MR may rarely be necessary for evaluation of the DRUJ in difficult cases.

Management

Complications include the following:

▶ Chronic disability if disruption of the DRUJ goes unnoticed for >10 weeks.

▶ Anterior interosseous nerve (AIN) palsy may occur but is often overlooked because there is no sensory component; AIN is a purely motor nerve and a division of the median nerve. Injury causes paralysis of the flexor pollicis longus and flexor digitorum profundus of the index finger, resulting in inability to pinch using the thumb and index finger. MR may be of benefit for further evaluation of the nerve.

▶ Nonunion

Treatment: Adults require open reduction of the radius and the DRUJ with compression-plate-and-screw fixation. Closed reduction may lead to further disability secondary to prolonged ulnar abutment. Skeletally immature patients are typically treated with closed reduction and casting.

Further Readings

Mann FA, Wilson AJ, Gilula LA. Radiographic evaluation of the wrist: What does the hand surgeon want to know? *Radiology* 1992;*184*:15–24.

Resnick D, Goergen RG. Physical injury: Extraspinal sites. In Resnick D, ed. *Diagnosis of Bone and Joint Disorders*, 3rd ed. Philadelphia: WB Saunders, 1995:2736–2737.

History

▸ Elbow and forearm pain status post motor vehicle accident

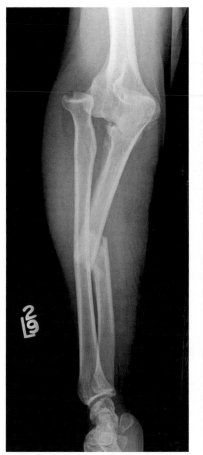

Figure 80.1

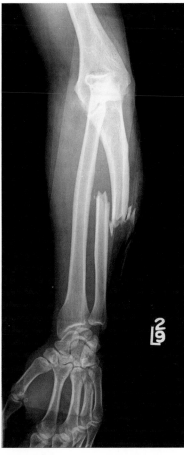

Figure 80.2

Case 80 Monteggia fracture-dislocation

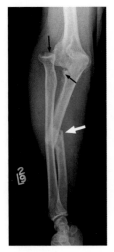
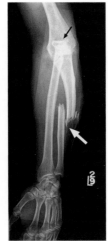

Figure 80.3   **Figure 80.4**

Findings

Figures 80.3 and 80.4 (AP and lateral radiographs of the left forearm) demonstrate a displaced fracture of the proximal ulnar diaphysis with anterior angulation (*white arrows*) in association with anterolateral dislocation of the radial head and widening of the proximal radial ulnar joint (*small black arrows*). The distal radial ulnar joint is intact.

Differential Diagnosis

None

Teaching Points

► Monteggia (ulnar metadiaphyseal fracture and radial head dislocation) and Galleazzi (distal radial diametaphyseal fracture and distal ulnar dislocation) are unstable injuries of the forearm.
► Evaluation of patients with ulnar or radial fractures must include the elbow and wrist so as to not miss a potential radial head dislocation (Monteggia fracture) or distal ulnar fracture (Galleazzi fracture).
► Mechanisms include direct blow and hyperpronation and hyperextension.
► Types of Monteggia fracture-dislocations
  1. Type 1 (extension type) (60%): anterior dislocation of the radial head (or fracture) and fracture of ulnar diaphysis with anterior angulation
  2. Type 2 (flexion type) (15%): posterior or posterolateral dislocation of the radial head (or fracture) and fracture of proximal ulnar diaphysis with posterior angulation
  3. Type 3 (20%): lateral or anterolateral dislocation of the radial head with fracture of the ulnar metaphysis
  4. Type 4 (5%): anterior dislocation of the radial head with fracture of the proximal third radius and ulna

Management

It is important to make the correct diagnosis because complications can include posterior interosseous nerve (PIN) palsy, radiohumeral ankylosis, recurrent radial head dislocation, nonunion of the ulnar fracture, and myositis ossificans. MR may be required to rule out annular tear and potential PIN impingement.

Further Readings

Resnick D, Goergen T. Physical injury: Extraspinal sites. In Resnick D, ed. *Diagnosis of Bone and Joint Disorders*, 4th ed. Philadelphia: WB Saunders2002: 2772–2734.

History

▶ Right shoulder pain

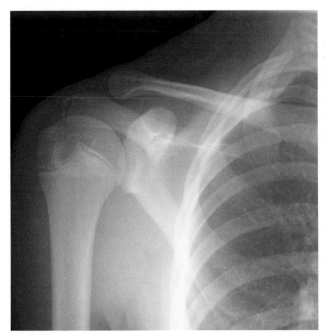

Figure 81.1

Case 81 Stress fracture, right first rib

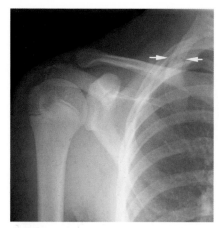

Figure 81.2

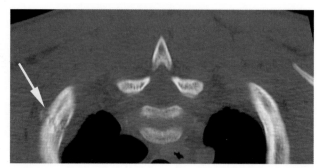

Figure 81.3

Findings

Figure 81.2 (AP view of the shoulder) demonstrates a nondisplaced fracture through the lateral aspect of the right first rib (*arrows*). Figure 81.3 (oblique axial reconstructed image from a CT of the chest) shows the fracture and early callus formation (*arrow*).

Differential Diagnosis

None

Teaching Points

- ▸ Stress fractures of the first rib occur most commonly in throwing athletes and may involve either their throwing or nonthrowing sides.
- ▸ These typically involve the lateral aspect of the rib, where the upward pull of the scalene muscles is opposed by the downward pull of the serratus anterior and intercostal muscles, resulting in focal stresses within the bone.
- ▸ Since these patients often present with "shoulder" pain, the fracture is easily overlooked on standard shoulder radiographs.

Management

Rest and a gradual return to throwing is often sufficient; however, a longer period of convalescence may be needed in cases of a complete fracture.

Further Readings

Coris EE, Higgins W II. First rib stress fractures in throwing athletes. *Am J Sports Med* 2005;33:1400–1404.

History

► 23-year-old man with shoulder pain following a seizure

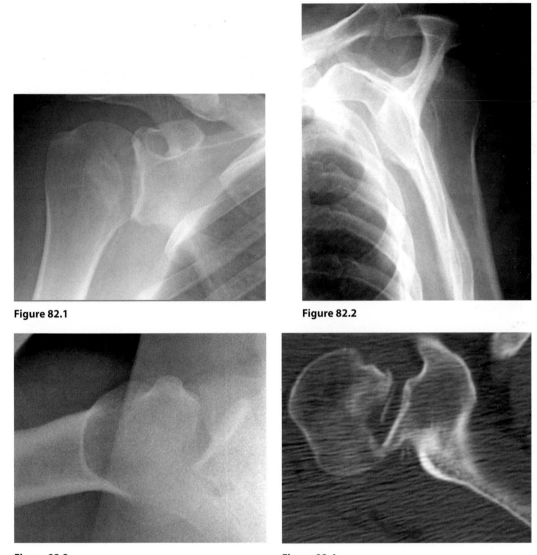

Figure 82.1

Figure 82.2

Figure 82.3

Figure 82.4

Case 82 Posterior shoulder dislocation

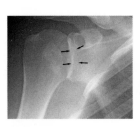 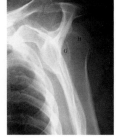 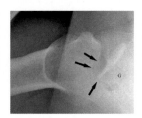 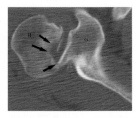

Figure 82.5   **Figure 82.6**   **Figure 82.7**   **Figure 82.8**

Findings

Figure 82.5 (AP radiograph of the right shoulder) demonstrates loss of the normal glenohumeral joint space with apparent overlap and second cortical line "trough sign" at the supramedial humeral head (*black arrows*). Figures 82.6 (scapular Y view) and 82.7 (axillary view) show posterior positioning of the humeral head with respect to the glenoid (G) with cortical impaction (reverse Hill Sachs) of the humeral head (H) on the posterior glenoid (*black arrows*) better shown on axial CT (Fig. 82.8) with multiple associated displaced cortical fragments.

Differential Diagnosis

Pathognomonic for posterior shoulder dislocation

Teaching Points

- ▶ Shoulder dislocations: 95% anterior, <5% posterior
- ▶ Posterior dislocation causes: seizures (may present with bilateral posterior shoulder dislocations), electrocution, electric shock therapy. Types: subacromial, subglenoid, and subspinous.
- ▶ Radiographs diagnostic:
  - ▪ AP shoulder demonstrates abnormal loss of the normal parallel appearance of the glenoid and humeral head, as in this case (unlike the antero-inferomedial positioning of the humeral head in anterior dislocation).
  - ▪ "Trough" sign (fixed internal rotation of the humerus with a second cortical line parallel and lateral to the humeral subchondral articular surface from impaction)
  - ▪ "Vacant" glenoid (space between the glenoid rim and humeral head often >6 mm)
  - ▪ Posterior humeral head positioning with respect to glenoid on scapular Y view and axillary views. The latter may demonstrates the potential reverse Hill-Sachs deformity of the humeral head related to impaction on the posterior glenoid during dislocation, which is better visualized on CT imaging.

Management

Relocation as per imaging status. Secondary osteoarthritis is a common complication if there is a delay in diagnosis and treatment. MRI may be of benefit to assess labral or soft tissue injuries that may require surgical intervention.

Further Readings

Gor DM. The trough line sign. *Radiology* 2002;*224*:485–486.
Resnick D, Goergen TG. Physical injury: Extraspinal sites. In *Diagnosis of Bone and Joint Disorders*, 3rd ed. Philadelphia, WB Saunders, 1995;2693–2824.

History

▶ 40-year-old man with severe neck pain status post recent motor vehicle accident

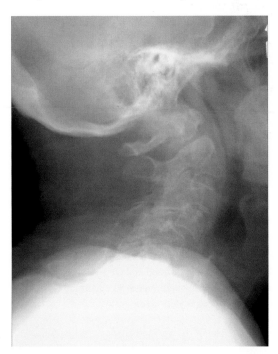

Figure 83.1

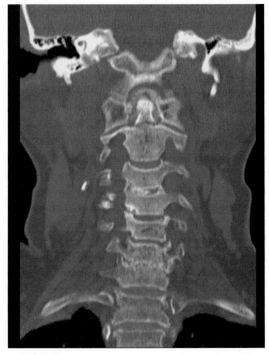

Figure 83.2

Case 83   Type 2 odontoid fracture

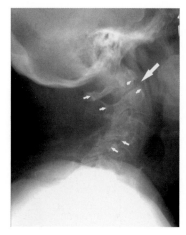
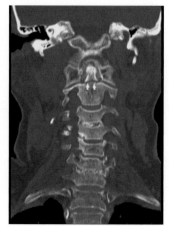

Figure 83.3   **Figure 83.4**

Findings

Figure 83.3 (lateral cervical spine radiograph) depicts a transverse fracture through the base of the odontoid at the C2 body junction (*white arrow*) with mild posterior subluxation of the odontoid and C1 arch with respect to C2 (*small arrows*). Grade 1 retrolisthesis of C5 on C4 is present (*small arrows*). Figure 83.4 (coronal CT) best demonstrates the linear lucent fracture through the base of the dens (*small white arrows*).

Differential Diagnosis

Pathognomonic, but congenital nonfusion of ossification centers may have this appearance and should be excluded, particularly in nontrauma patients.

Teaching Points

► Odontoid fractures constitute 15% of all cervical spine fractures and are usually secondary to motor vehicle accidents or falls.
► Mechanism of injury includes a combination of flexion, extension, and rotation.
► Three primary types listed below are better evaluated with multidetector CT:
  ▪ Type 1 (tip of odontoid)—stable
  ▪ Type 2 (base of odontoid)—unstable
  ▪ Type 3 (through the body of the axis)—may be stable or unstable
► Associated injuries such as C1 anterior ring fractures (Jefferson burst fracture) are relatively common, and a prevertebral soft tissue thickening of >10 mm on plain films is highly suggestive.

Management

Cervical radiographs are performed first, with CT typically utilized for further characterization of the extent or number of fractures. MR imaging is useful for further evaluation of ligamentous or soft tissue injury that may occur in conjunction with these injuries. While internal fixation is often recommended in patients, particularly with offset, the best surgical treatment for type 2 fractures of the dens is still controversial.

Further Readings

Denaro V, Papalia R, Di Martino A, Denaro L, Maffulli N. The best surgical treatment for type II fractures of the dens is still controversial. *Clin Orthop Relat Res* 2011;469(3):742–750.

Rao SK, Wasyliw C, Nunez DB. Spectrum of imaging findings in hyperextension injuries of the neck. *Radiographics* 2005;25(5):1239–1254.

History

▶ Trauma

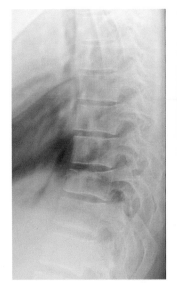

Figure 84.1

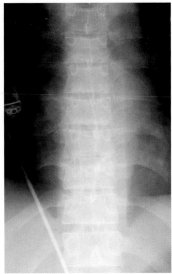

Figure 84.2

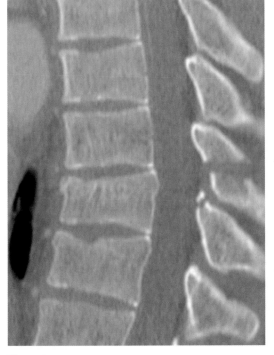

Figure 84.3

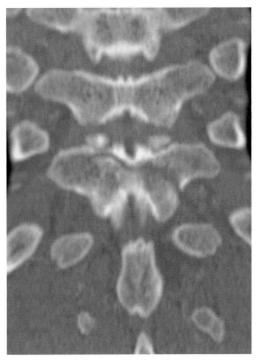

Figure 84.4

Case 84 Flexion-distraction ("Chance") fracture

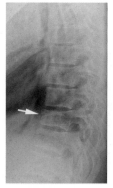

Figure 84.5

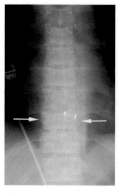

Figure 84.6

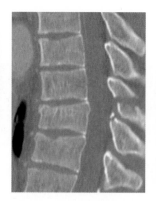

Figure 84.7

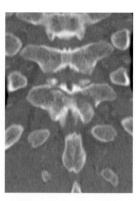

Figure 84.8

Findings

Lateral (Fig. 84.5) and AP (Fig. 84.6) views of the thoracic spine demonstrate anterior wedging of the T10 vertebrae (*arrows*). Sagittal (Fig. 84.7) and coronal (Fig. 84.8) reformatted CT images show that the fracture not only involves the vertebral body but extends through the posterior elements as well. Note that the posterior element involvement is evident but less easily characterized on the AP radiograph (*arrowheads*).

Differential Diagnosis

Simple compression fracture; burst fracture

Teaching Points

- ▶ Fractures of the thoracic spine are usually secondary to high-energy trauma and most commonly involve the vertebrae around the thoracolumbar junction.
- ▶ Classically, the vertebrae are divided into three "columns" for grading purposes: anterior (anterior two thirds of the body), middle (posterior third of the body), and posterior (all elements posterior to the vertebral body).
- ▶ Fractures occur along a spectrum and include the following:
  - – Simple compression: involves the anterior column only
  - – Burst: involves anterior and middle columns
  - – Flexion-distraction: involves all three columns
  - – Fracture-dislocation: the most severe type, usually results in cord injury
- ▶ A flexion-distraction injury (also known as a "Chance" or "lapbelt" fracture) results from severe tensile forces that essentially "pull" the spine apart. Disruption may extend through bone and/or soft tissues (disk, ligaments).
- ▶ These are easily misdiagnosed as simple compression or burst fractures because the posterior-element involvement is easily missed on radiographs. As such, CT has assumed a larger role in evaluating thoracolumbar fractures.

Management

These are unstable injuries and require surgical stabilization.

Further Readings

Bernstein MP, Mirvis SE, Shanmuganathan K. Chance-type fractures of the thoracolumbar spine: imaging analysis in 53 patients. *AJR Am J Roentgenol* 2006;*187*:859–868.

History

▸ 15-year-old boy with left hip pain

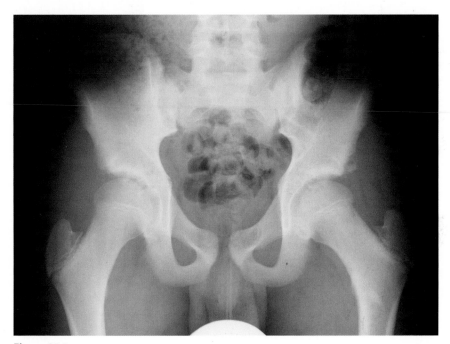

Figure 85.1

Case 85   Avulsion fracture, anterior inferior iliac spine

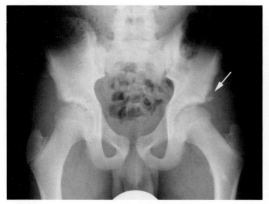

Figure 85.2

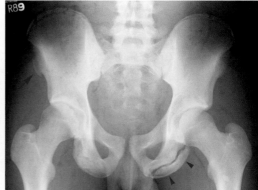

Figure 85.3

Findings

Figure 85.2 (AP view of the pelvis) demonstrates an avulsion fracture of the left anterior inferior iliac spine (*arrow*), the site of origin of the rectus femoris tendon. Figure 85.3 (AP view of the pelvis in the same patient 3 years later [at age 18]) shows evidence of subacute/chronic avulsion fractures of the left ischial tuberosity and inferior pubic ramus (*arrowheads*) and right anterior superior iliac spine (*arrow*).

Differential Diagnosis

None

Teaching Points

▶ Avulsion fractures are most common in young patients owing to the fact that muscle strength outpaces skeletal development during adolescence, and the unfused physis is the weak link in the muscle-tendon-bone unit.
  ▪ Affected sites around the pelvis and proximal femur include the following:
  ▪ Common: anterior superior iliac spine (sartorius, tensor fascia lata), anterior inferior iliac spine (rectus femoris), ischial tuberosity (common hamstring tendon)
  ▪ Uncommon: iliac crest (abdominal wall muscles), parasymphyseal (rectus abdominis), lesser tuberosity of the femur (iliopsoas)

Management

Conservative, supportive therapy

Further Readings

Rossi F, Dragoni S. Acute avulsion fractures of the pelvis in adolescent competitive athletes: prevalence, location and sports distribution of 203 cases collected. *Skeletal Radiol* 2001;*30*:127–131.

History

▶ History of ankle trauma with persistent pain

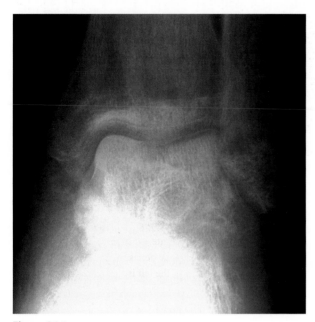

Figure 86.1

Case 86   Segmental avascular necrosis of the talus after fracture (partial Hawkins sign)

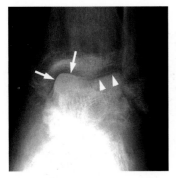

Figure 86.2

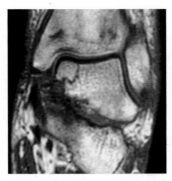

Figure 86.3

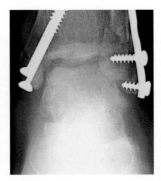

Figure 86.4

Findings

Figure 86.2 (AP radiograph of the ankle several weeks after trauma) reveals severe diffuse osteopenia throughout the bones of the ankle with the exception of the medial talar dome (*arrows*) compatible with an area of segmental avascular necrosis (absence of a normal Hawkins sign). Note the normal Hawkins sign (subchondral lucency) along the lateral talar dome (*arrowheads*). Figure 86.3 (coronal T1-weighted image of the ankle) shows a low-signal fracture line through that corner of the talar dome. Figure 86.4 (AP radiograph of the ankle in a different patient) demonstrates a normal Hawkins sign along the entire talar dome.

Differential Diagnosis

None

Teaching Points

- ▶ The Hawkins sign is a thin subchondral rim of lucency seen along the talar dome 8 to 12 weeks after an ankle injury. It is a normal phenomenon, related to the osteoclastic resorption that produces the osteopenia seen with disuse.
- ▶ Disruption of the blood supply to all or a portion of the talar dome results in absence of the Hawkins sign (subchondral sclerosis), which usually indicates underlying avascular necrosis.

Management

Potential curettage and grafting of the affected portion of the talar dome

Further Readings

Tehranzadeh J, Stuffman E, Ross SDK. Partial Hawkins sign in fractures of the talus: a report of three cases. *AJR Am J Roentgenol* 2003;*181*:1559–1563.

Tezval M, Dumont C, Sturmer KM. Prognostic reliability of the Hawkins sign in fractures of the talus. *J Orthop Trauma* 2007;*21*:538–543.

History

▸ Injury to foot.

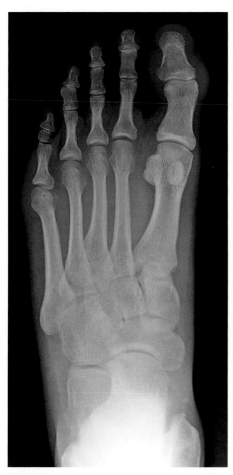

Figure 87.1

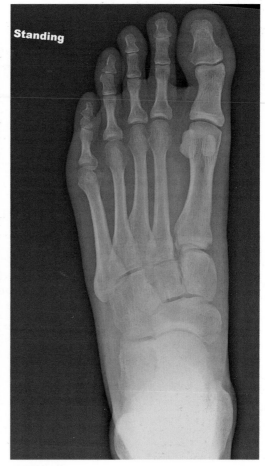

Standing

Figure 87.2

Case 87 Lisfranc injury

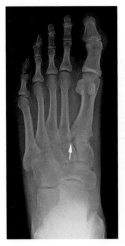
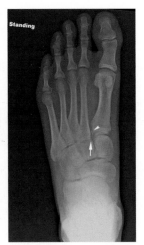

Figure 87.3   **Figure 87.4**

Findings

Figure 87.3 (AP [non-weightbearing] radiograph of the foot) demonstrates subtle lateral displacement of the base of the second metatarsal relative to the middle cuneiform (*arrow*). This is better demonstrated on a weightbearing view (Fig. 87.4, *arrow*), as is an associated fracture involving the base of the first metatarsal (*arrowhead*).

Differential Diagnosis

None

Teaching Points

- ▶ The five tarsal-metatarsal joints are collectively known as the "Lisfranc" joint.
- ▶ The Lisfranc ligament extends from the lateral aspect of the medial cuneiform to the medial margin of the base of the second metatarsal and is a crucial stabilizer of the midfoot.
- ▶ Early and accurate diagnosis of a traumatic disruption of the Lisfranc ligament is important because misdiagnosis can result in long-term midfoot instability and a poor outcome. However, these injuries are often missed on initial radiographs, especially if not obtained with weightbearing.
- ▶ Radiographic signs of Lisfranc injury include lateral displacement of the base of the second metatarsal relative to the medial margin of the middle cuneiform on an AP view, widening of the space between the proximal aspects of the first and second metatarsals, and small cortical fractures in that region.
- ▶ Weightbearing views with or without craniocaudal angulation may better demonstrate the alignment abnormalities, as illustrated in this case.
- ▶ CT provides better delineation of these injuries, especially if there is a high degree of clinical suspicion despite normal-appearing radiographs.

Management

Nondisplaced Lisfranc injuries may be treated with immobilization, but surgical fixation is often required, especially in those cases with clear dislocation and/or significant displacement.

Further Readings

Rankine JJ, Nicholas CM, Wells G, Barron DA. The diagnostic accuracy of radiogrphs in Lisfranc injury and the potential value of a craniocaudal projection. *AJR Am J Roentgenol* 2012;*198*:W365–369.

History

▶ Right hip pain without history of recent injury

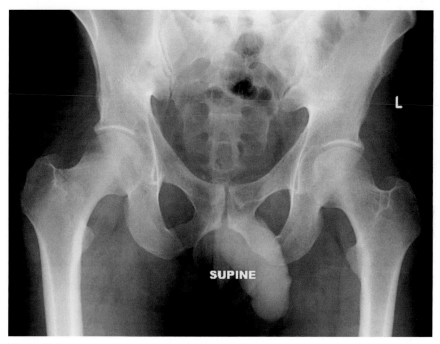

Figure 88.1

Case 88 Developing stress fracture of the right femoral neck (lateral aspect)

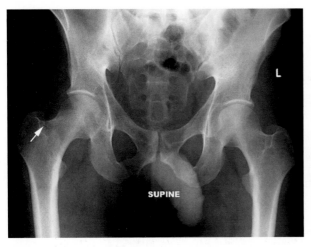

Figure 88.2

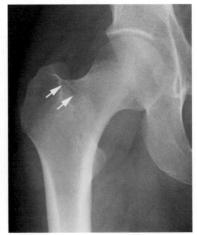

Figure 88.3

Findings

Figure 88.2 (AP radiograph of the pelvis) demonstrates a subtle, incomplete fracture line involving the lateral femoral neck (*arrow*) that is better seen in a magnified image (Fig. 88.3, *arrows*).

Differential Diagnosis

None

Teaching Points

▶ Stress fractures are typically divided into "fatigue" and "insufficiency" types (resulting from increased stresses placed on normal bone or normal stresses applied to abnormal bone, respectively).

▶ Stress injuries are most common in the lower extremities, and typical sites include the femoral neck, tibial shaft, calcaneus, navicular, and metatarsals.

▶ Those in certain locations are considered "high risk" because of their propensity to displace and/or demonstrate poor healing. These include the lateral femoral neck, anterior tibial shaft, tarsal navicular, and fifth metatarsal.

▶ The convex lateral margin of the proximal femur experiences strong tensile forces with weightbearing that will tend to distract the margins of a developing stress fracture in that region and result in a displaced fracture.

▶ Fortunately, stress fractures occur more commonly along the concave medial femoral neck, where compressive forces result in better fracture healing and less risk of complication.

Management

While stress fractures along the medial femoral neck can be treated conservatively, those involving the lateral neck are usually pinned prophylactically to avoid a displaced fracture, as discussed above.

Further Readings

Boden BP, Osbahr DC. High-risk stress fractures: evaluation and treatment. *J Am Acad Orthop Surg* 2000;8:344–353.

History

► Ankle injury

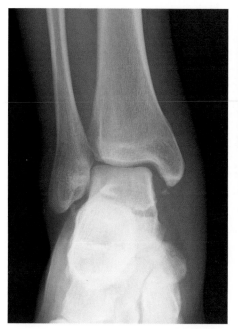

Figure 89.1

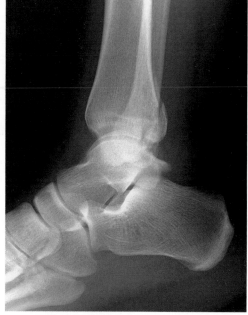

Figure 89.2

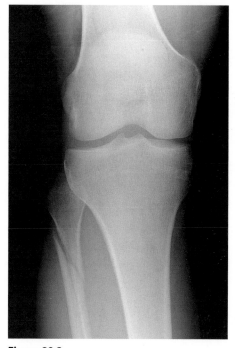

Figure 89.3

Case 89 Maisonneuve injury

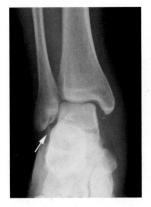

Figure 89.4

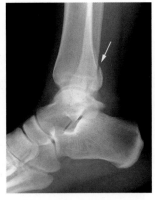

Figure 89.5

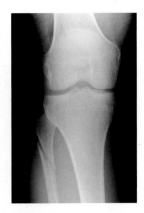

Figure 89.6

Findings

Figure 89.4 (AP view of the ankle) demonstrates a small fracture at the tip of the medial malleolus, widening of the medial mortise, and distal tibiofibular syndesmosis as well as a probable fracture fragment adjacent to the tip of the lateral malleolus as well (*arrow*). Figure 89.5 (lateral view of the ankle) shows a minimally displaced fracture of the posterior malleolus (*arrow*). Figure 89.6 (AP view of the right knee) reveals an oblique fracture of the proximal fibular shaft (Maisonneuve injury).

Differential Diagnosis

None

Teaching Points

▶ Complex ankle injuries result in a variety of bone and ligament pathology.
▶ As in this case, radiographs often demonstrate fractures, and abnormalities in alignment are secondary clues to associated ligamentous injuries.
▶ Injury to the distal tibiofibular syndesmosis is also known as a "high ankle sprain" and typically results from external rotation of the talus that produces a fracture of the medial malleolus and/or rupture of the deltoid ligament.
▶ Further impaction of the talus against the lateral malleolus drives the fibula laterally, resulting in rupture of the anterior tibiofibular ligament and propagation of the force proximally through the interosseous ligament.
▶ This force often exits laterally, producing a fracture of the proximal fibula known as a Maisonneuve injury.
▶ Awareness of this injury pattern is important since the proximal fibular fracture may go undetected if only imaging of the ankle is performed and result in instability of the proximal tibiofibular joint. As a result, radiographs of the knee should be considered in patients with complex ankle injuries.

Management

Mild syndesmotic injuries may be treated nonoperatively, while more severe injuries are usually treated with internal fixation and, if needed, ligament reconstruction. The proximal fibular fracture will typically heal with immobilization.

Further Readings

Porter DA. Evaluation and treatment of ankle syndesmosis injuries. *AAOS Instr Course Lect* 2009;58:575–581.

History

▶ Trauma

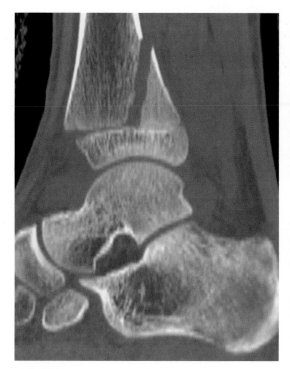

Figure 90.1

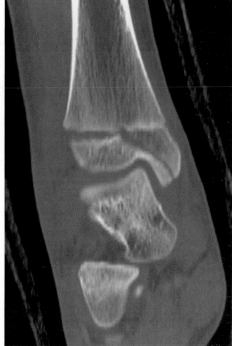

Figure 90.2

Case 90 Triplane fracture of the distal tibia

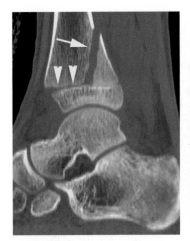

Figure 90.3

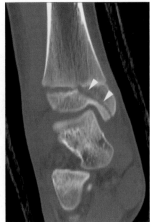

Figure 90.4

Findings

Figure 90.3 (sagittal reconstructed CT image of the ankle) demonstrates a coronally oriented fracture involving the posterior metaphysis (*arrow*) with an axially oriented component extending through the anterior physis (*arrowheads*). Figure 90.4 (coronal reconstructed CT image) reveals a third, sagitally oriented fracture line extending through the epiphysis (*arrowheads*).

Differential Diagnosis

None

Teaching Points

▶ A triplane fracture is a complex intra-articular fracture of the distal tibia that most commonly affects adolescent patients when the tibial growth plate has partially fused.

▶ As its name implies, fracture lines are seen in all three planes. The most common configuration involves a coronally oriented fracture of the posterior tibial metaphysis, an axially oriented fracture extending through the physis anterior to that level, and a sagitally oriented fracture involving the anterior epiphysis.

▶ While the posterior metaphyseal fracture is a Salter-Harris type II and the anterior epiphyseal fracture is a Salter-Harris type III, the combination of fracture lines constitutes a Salter-Harris type IV injury.

▶ Radiography is often diagnostic, although the exact fracture morphology and degree of fragment displacement will be better demonstrated with CT.

Management

Nondisplaced and extra-articular fractures may be treated with casting, but displaced fractures typically require open reduction and internal fixation

Further Readings

Brown SD, Kasser JR, Zurakowski D, Jaramillo D. Analysis of 51 tibial triplane fractures using CT with multiplanar reconstruction. *AJR Am J Roentgenol* 2004;*183*:1489–1495.

Schnetzler KA, Hoernschemeyer D. The pediatric triplane ankle fracture. *J Am Acad Orthop Surg* 2007;*15*:738–747.

History

▶ 80-year-old woman with right knee pain for 2 weeks after stepping off a porch

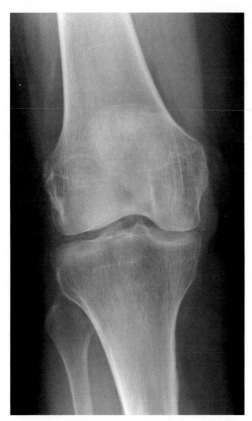

Figure 91.1

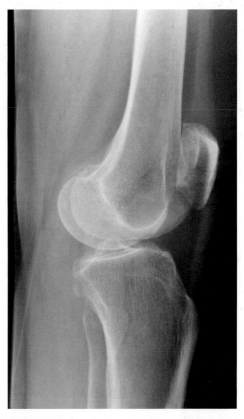

Figure 91.2

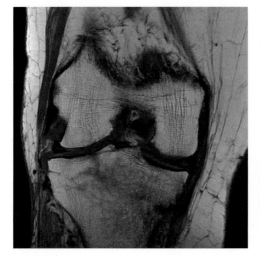

Figure 91.3

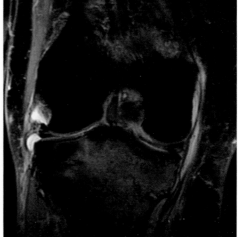

Figure 91.4

Case 91   Occult nondisplaced tibial plateau fracture

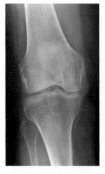
Figure 91.5

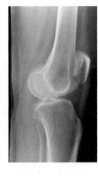
Figure 91.6

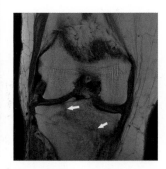
Figure 91.7

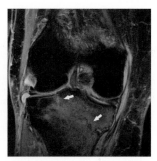
Figure 91.8

Findings

Figures 91.5 and 91.6 (initial AP and lateral right knee radiographs) demonstrate no evidence of abnormality. MRI performed one week later depicts an oblique supramedial nondisplaced tibial plateau fracture with a low intensity fracture line (*white arrows*) on Figures 91.7 (coronal T1) and 91.8 (coronal STIR) with surrounding bone marrow edema.

Differential Diagnosis

None

Teaching Points

▸ MR is much more sensitive than radiographs for detection of early fractures, with edema appearing early and a nondisplaced fracture line becoming better seen over time. Associated soft tissue injuries are better evaluated on MR.
▸ CT is useful for delineation of cortical extension and potential step or gap deformities.
▸ The Schatzker classification system of tibial plateau fractures reflects mechanism of injury and imaging pattern and helps determine treatment plan:
  ▪ Schatzker I—lateral split
  ▪ Schatzker II—split with depression
  ▪ Schatzker III—pure lateral depression
  ▪ Schatzker IV—pure medial depression
  ▪ Schatzker V—bicondylar
▸ Scintigraphy demonstrates increased uptake in the region of the fracture immediately but is not specific.
▸ Follow-up radiographs in 7 to 10 days usually demonstrate sclerosis due to reparative bone along the fracture line, confirming fracture.

Management

Conservative treatment and rest for occult nondisplaced fractures. Internal fixation may be required according to type of Schatzker injury, if step or gap deformity are noted on CT or if soft tissue derangements are noted on MR imaging that require surgical intervention. Radiographic follow-up should be performed to assess healing.

Further Readings

Berger P, Ofstein R, Jackson D, Morrison D, Silvino N, Amador R. MR demonstration of radiographically occult fractures: what have we been missing? *Radiographics* 1989;*9*(3):407–436.

May DA, Purins JL, Smith DK. MR imaging of occult traumatic fractures and muscular injuries of the hip and pelvis in elderly patients. *Am J Roentgenol* 1996;*166*:1075–1078.

History

▶ 82-year-old woman on bisphosphonate therapy with intermittent proximal thigh pain

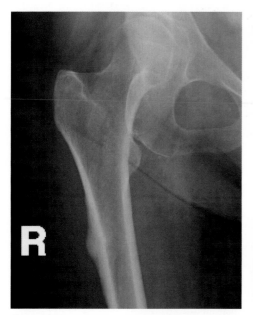

Figure 92.1

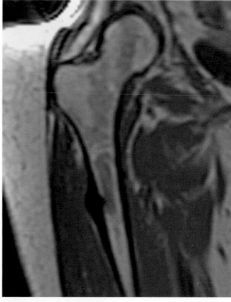

Figure 92.2

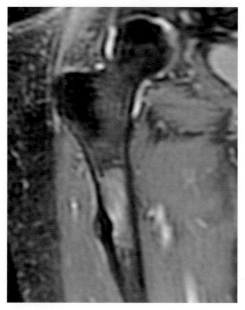

Figure 92.3

Case 92 Chronic insufficiency fracture (bisphosphonate-related)

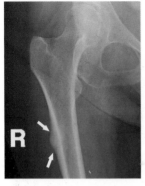

Figure 92.4

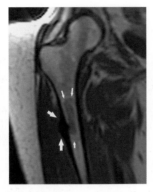

Figure 92.5

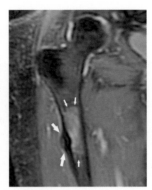

Figure 92.6

Findings

Figure 92.4 (AP radiograph of the right femur) demonstrates proximal lateral beaklike cortical thickening (*white arrows on all images*). Figures 92.5 and 92.6 (coronal T1-weighted and STIR MR images) confirm persistent low-signal-intensity beaklike lateral proximal femoral cortical thickening with endosteal and periosteal edema (low T1 and high STIR) (*small arrows*), confirming a healing stress fracture.

Differential Diagnosis

Pathognomonic but could consider: chronic infection of cortex; osteoid osteoma (child)

Teaching Points

▶ Atypical transverse or oblique proximal lateral or subtrochanteric cortical fractures of the femoral diaphysis with "beaking" of the cortex and diffuse cortical thickening of the proximal shaft have been shown to be characteristic of bisphosphonate-related chronic insufficiency fractures

▶ Bisphosphonate insufficiency fractures ("Fosamax fractures") typically occur in postmenopausal osteoporotic women on alendronate treatment for >5 years following little or noncharacteristic minor trauma.

▶ Bisphosphonates act on osteoclasts to inhibit bone resorption, initially increasing bone mineral density and strength within the first 5 years of treatment and preventing vertebral and femoral neck fractures in postmenopausal osteoporotic women. However longer term therapy (>5 years) leads to decreased strength of bone at areas of high tensile stress, particularly the subtrochanteric and diaphyseal regions of the femur where repetitive microtrabecular injury results in insufficiency fractures.

▶ Most patients have a prodrome of thigh pain, vague discomfort, or weakness.

Management

Radiographs of the femur are recommended in any patient with thigh pain on bisphosphonates. Contralateral femoral imaging is performed in patients with known complete fractures because cortical thickening or fractures have been shown in the other femur in some patients. MR, CT, and bone scan can help detect early stress changes or incomplete fractures. Although drug holidays have been recommended, they have not been proven to prevent fractures. Treatment is surgical fixation or prophylactic pinning.

Further Readings

Lenart BA, Lorich DG, Lane JM. Atypical fractures of the femoral diaphysis in postmenopausal women taking alendronate. *N Engl J Med* 2008;*358*(12):1304–1306.

Porrino JA, Kohl CA, Taljanovic M, Rogers LF. Diagnosis of proximal femoral insufficiency fractures in patients receiving bisphosphonate therapy. *AJR Am J Roentgenol* 2010;*194*(4):1061–1064.

History

▶ 32-year-old female marathon runner with severe anterior calf pain

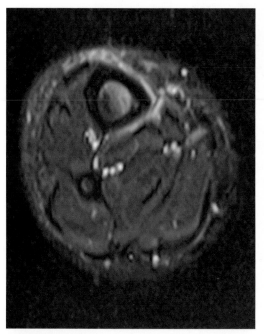

Figure 93.1

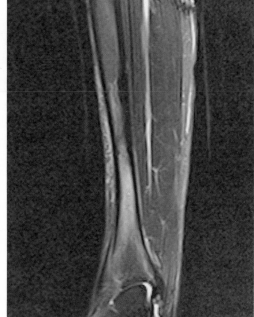

Figure 93.2

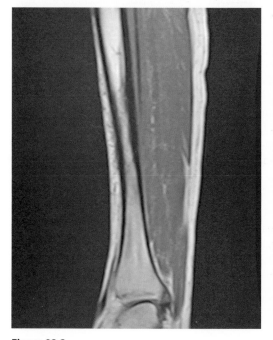

Figure 93.3

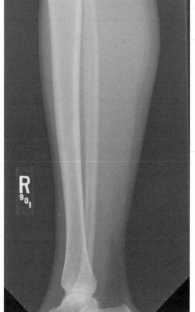

Figure 93.4

Case 93 Tibial stress reaction (grade 3/5)

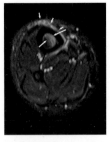 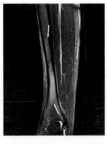 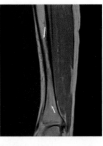 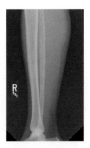

Figure 93.5   **Figure 93.6**   **Figure 93.7**   **Figure 93.8**

Findings

Figure 93.5 (axial T2-weighted FS image of the right mid-distal calf) demonstrates anteromedial periosteal edema (*small arrows*) paralleling the tibial cortex with associated intramedullary tibial marrow edema (*arrows*) without cortical involvement or linear fracture line. Figure 93.6 (sagittal STIR MR image) confirms abnormal high signal intensity within the tibial marrow (*arrow*) with corresponding decreased signal intensity on the sagittal T1-weighted image, Figure 93.7 (*arrows*). Figure 93.8 (lateral radiograph of the right tibia) demonstrates no evidence of fracture or new bone formation. Incidental calcification of the anterior distal subcutaneous tissues is seen.

Differential Diagnosis

Infection (osteomyelitis) or contusion; normal nutrient vessel (thin and tubular) or marrow hyperplasia; neoplastic infiltration (lymphoma)

Teaching Points

- Stress injuries are common following excessive use, particularly in athletes, and often have a nonspecific clinical presentation. Not all stress injuries are symptomatic.
- Common locations: tibia (anterior: mid-distal shaft; posterior: junction of proximal and middle third or distal and middle third), metatarsals, femoral neck, sesamoids, navicular, calcaneus, patella, pelvis.
- Radiographs are typically insensitive unless chronic bone formation or linear fracture is present.
- Tc99 bone scan has high sensitivity and demonstrates abnormal activity earlier than radiographic changes appear, but suffers from poor specificity.
- MR is the study of choice, with high sensitivity and specificity.
- Five-stage MR grading system (parallels bone scan findings):
  - 0: Normal study
  - 1: Subtle periosteal edema on T2 FS or STIR (commonly along the anteromedial surface of the tibia.)
  - 2: Periosteal edema and increased marrow signal on T2 FS with subtle low signal on T1
  - 3: More extensive periosteal edema with marrow signal abnormalities visible on T2 and T1 images
  - 4: Abnormal signal within the cortex and/or discrete fracture line
- The term "shin splints" is a non-specific clinical description of lower leg pain that may or may not correlate with MR imaging abnormalities.

Management

Early diagnosis and accurate grading of the injury by imaging is critical to implement appropriate management and treatment, prevent progression of injury, and allow return to activity. Severity progresses with stage, as does time to recovery.

Further Readings

Bergman AG, Fredericson M, Ho C, Matheson GO. Asymptomatic tibial stress reactions: MRI detection and clinical follow-up in long-distance runners. *AJR Am J Roentgenol* 2004;*183*(3):635–638.

Hwang B, Fredericson M, Chung CB, Beaulier CF, Gold GE. MRI findings of femoral diaphyseal stress injuries in athletes. *AJR Am J Roentgenol* 2005;*185*(1):166–173.

Pavlov H. Physical injury: Sports-related abnormalities. In Resnick D, ed. *Diagnosis of Bone and Joint Disorders*, 3rd ed. Philadelphia: WB Saunders, 1995:3229–3263.

History

▶ Pain after knee injury

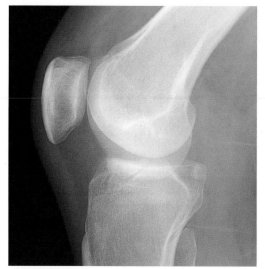

Figure 94.1

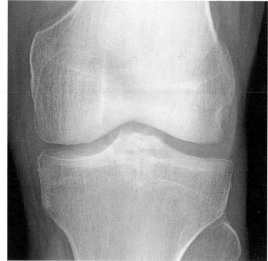

Figure 94.2

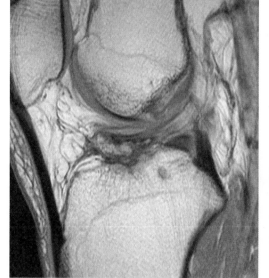

Figure 94.3

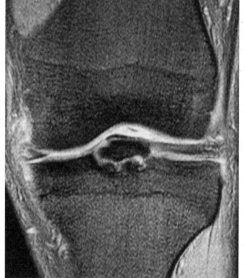

Figure 94.4

Case 94 Avulsion fracture of the tibial plateau at the attachment of the anterior cruciate ligament

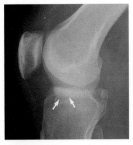

Figure 94.5

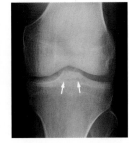

Figure 94.6

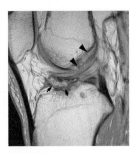

Figure 94.7

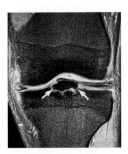

Figure 94.8

Findings

Figure 94.5 (lateral radiograph of the knee) demonstrates a faint curvilinear lucency involving the anterior tibial plateau (*arrows*). Figure 94.6 (AP radiograph) reveals that the lucency involves the central plateau at the level of the tibial spines (*arrows*). Sagittal proton density (Fig. 94.7) and coronal (Fig. 94.8) gradient echo images reveal the lucency to represent an avulsion fracture (*arrows*) at the tibial attachment of the anterior cruciate ligament (ACL—*arrowheads* in Fig. 94.7)

Differential Diagnosis

None

Teaching Points

▶ Radiographic signs of an ACL injury include a "deep notch" sign, a Segond fracture, and an avulsion fracture along the anterior tibial plateau, as in this case.

▶ The fracture typically involves the tibial spines and is more often seen in younger, skeletally immature patients.

▶ It is important to report the size of the avulsed fragment of bone, because if it is large enough, and the ACL itself is intact, the bone fragment may be reattached to the plateau, thereby obviating the need for an ACL reconstruction.

Management

Surgical fixation of the fracture fragment if it is large enough; ACL reconstruction if the fragment is small or comminuted

Further Readings

Prince JS, Laor T, Bean JA. MRI of anterior cruciate ligament injuries and associated findings in the pediatric knee: changes with skeletal maturation. *AJR Am J Roentgenol* 2005;*185*:756–762.

History

▸ 13-year-old boy with knee pain after an injury

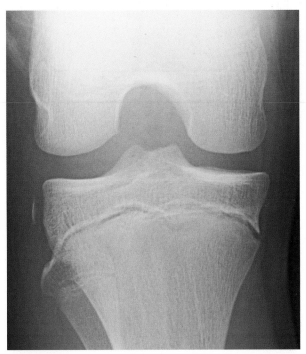

Figure 95.1

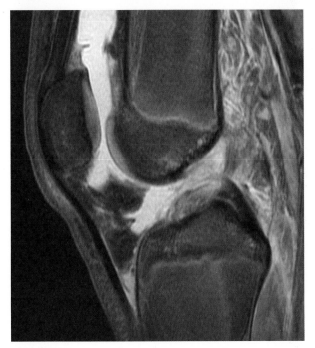

Figure 95.2

Case 95 Segond fracture and anterior cruciate ligament tear

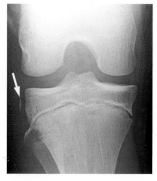
Figure 95.3

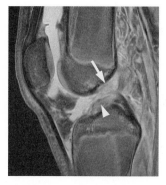
Figure 95.4

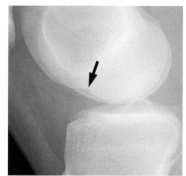
Figure 95.5

Findings

Figure 95.3 (AP radiograph) reveals a small avulsion fracture along the lateral tibial plateau (Segond fracture, *arrow*). Figure 95.4 (sagittal fat-saturated T2-weighted image) demonstrates a complete tear of the anterior cruciate ligament (ACL) near its femoral attachment (*arrow*). Note the lax fibers of the torn ligament (*arrowhead*). Figure 95.5 (lateral radiograph of the knee in another patient with an ACL tear) demonstrates a "deep sulcus sign" along the lateral femoral condyle (*arrow*). This sign is diagnosed when the lateral sulcus (which is normally present at that site on the condyle) measures >2 mm in depth. This finding results from the impaction forces that commonly occur in the lateral compartment with an ACL tear.

Differential Diagnosis

None

Teaching Points

▶ The ACL is most commonly torn when the foot is planted and the femur externally rotates relative to the tibia. Typically, the knee then buckles, with a valgus force that results in impaction injuries in the lateral femorotibial compartment.

▶ Disruption of the normally taut ligament can be directly observed with MR imaging, but there are also secondary radiographic findings that can be associated with an ACL tear.

▶ A Segond fracture, as in this case, results from avulsion of the posterior fibers of the iliotibial tract along the lateral margin of the tibial plateau from the capsule. While only 10% of patients with ACL tears demonstrate a Segond fracture, an ACL tear is found in 75% to 100% of those patients who demonstrate this finding.

▶ Other secondary radiographic findings of an ACL tear include a "deep sulcus sign," avulsion of the tibial spines, and uncommonly avulsion of the fibular head ("arcuate sign").

Management

Surgical reconstruction of the ACL is commonly performed in these cases.

Further Readings

Garth WP Jr, Greco J, House MA. The lateral notch sign associated with acute anterior cruciate ligament disruption. *Am J Sports Med* 2000;*28*:68–73.

Gottsegen CJ, Eyer BA, White EA, Learch TJ, Forrester D. Avulsion fractures of the knee: imaging findings and clinical significance. *Radiographics* 2008;*28*:1755–1770.

History

▶ Elderly patient with symptoms of central cord syndrome after trauma

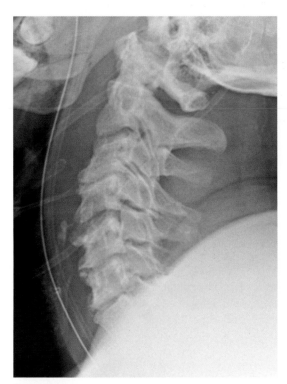

Figure 96.1

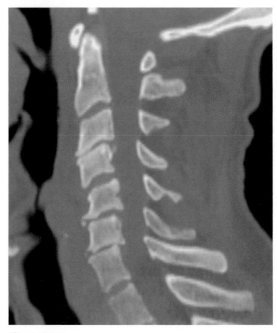

Figure 96.2

Case 96 Hyperextension injury

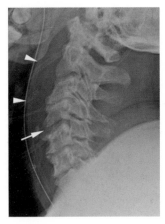

Figure 96.3

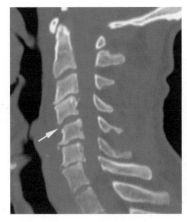

Figure 96.4

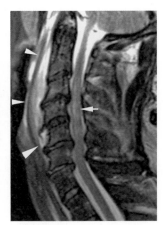

Figure 96.5

Findings

Figures 96.3 (lateral radiograph) and 96.4 (sagittal reformatted CT image of the cervical spine) demonstrate prominent prevertebral soft tissue swelling (*arrowheads* in Fig. 96.3), advanced multilevel spondylosis, and relative widening of the C4–5 disk space (*arrows*). Figure 96.5 (sagittal fat-saturated T2-weighted image) shows the prevertebral fluid/hemorrhage (*small arrowheads*) as well as disruption of the anterior longitudinal ligament at the C4–5 level (*large arrowhead*) and abnormal edema-like signal within the spinal cord at this level (*arrow*).

Differential Diagnosis

Radiograph and CT: cervical spondylosis without fracture. MRI: none.

Teaching Points

► A hyperextension force applied to the head (such as when the chin is struck during a fall) may result in transient posterior subluxation of the cervical vertebrae, producing injuries to the supporting soft tissues and spinal cord. These types of injuries are especially common in older patients.

► The cord injury is often the result of transient compression of the cord from posterior osteophytes or a thickened posterior longitudinal ligament (usually present in this age group), producing a "central cord syndrome" in which symptoms are more pronounced in the upper than lower extremities.

► Radiographs often underestimate the degree of injury because the vertebrae return to normal alignment without resulting in a fracture. Radiographic findings that should raise the suspicion of this injury include prominent anterior soft tissue swelling and focal widening of a single disk space.

► MR is diagnostic as it is able to display the associated soft tissue injuries, which may include prevertebral edema/hemorrhage, disruption of the anterior longitudinal ligament, disruption of an intervertebral disk, and edema or hemorrhage within the adjacent spinal cord.

Management

Supportive therapy and surgical decompression and stabilization

Further Readings

Rao SK, Wasyliw C, Nunez DB. Spectrum of imaging findings in hyperextension injuries of the neck. *Radiographics* 2005;*25*:1239–1254.

History

▶ 46-year-old woman with chronic radicular back pain

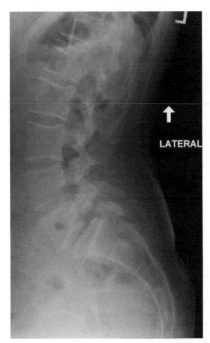

Figure 97.1

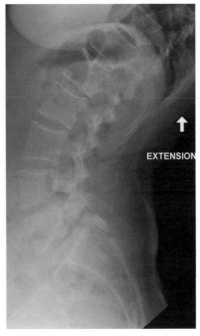

Figure 97.2

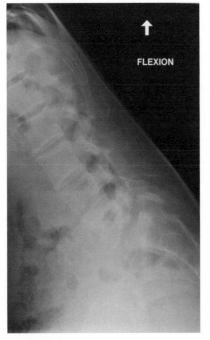

Figure 97.3

Case 97   Spondylolysis and spondylolisthesis L5/S1 due to pars interarticularis defects

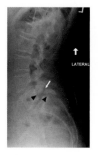

Figure 97.4

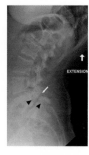

Figure 97.5

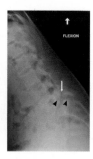

Figure 97.6

Findings

Lateral (Fig. 97.4), extension (Fig. 97.5), and flexion (Fig. 97.6) lumbosacral spine radiographs demonstrate a lucent oblique defect of the pars interarticularis (spondylolysis) at L5-S1 (*white arrows*) with grade 1 anterior spondylolisthesis of L5 on S1 (*black arrowheads*). There is no abnormal motion between flexion/extension views to suggest instability.

Differential Diagnosis

Posttraumatic versus congenital pars defects

Teaching Points

- ▶ Pars interarticularis defect (spondylolysis) is a visible interruption of the vertebral arch between the superior and inferior articular processes (pars articularis).
- ▶ Location: L5 (82%) > L4 (14%); rarely L3 (1%)
- ▶ Cause: Congenital or acquired (trauma), present in 4% to 6% of general population, commonly active young people (particularly gymnasts). Often bilateral but can be unilateral.
- ▶ Spondylolisthesis (abnormal slippage of vertebral body with relation to adjacent vertebra) is present in 80% of cases, the majority with bilateral spondylolysis.
- ▶ Spondylolisthesis is graded from 1 to 4 (Grade 1: quarter body uncovered; Grade 2: half body uncovered, etc.).
- ▶ Abnormal pars articularis lucency on lateral radiographs with (chronic) or without (acute) sclerosis. Oblique radiographs are most sensitive depicting the characteristic lucency through the "Scotty dog" neck.
- ▶ Instability (abnormal increased motion at the level of involvement) is best assessed with flexion/extension radiographs.
- ▶ Multiplanar CT can confirm bilateral involvement and extent and determine acute versus chronic nature. MR and Bone Scan demonstrate increased signal/activity at the area of involvement.

Management

MR imaging and radionuclide bone scans are useful for differentiating pars injuries for other entities and directing further treatment. Conservative treatment is appropriate if there is no instability or symptoms. Internal fixation is indicated if there is significant spondylolisthesis and pain, or instability. Addition of a bone growth stimulator in difficult cases has shown promise.

Further Readings

Camilo J, Jimenez M, Shabshin N, Laor N, Jaramillo D. Taking the stress out of evaluating stress injuries in children. *Radiographics* 2012;*32*(2):537–555.

McTimoney CA, Micheli LJ. Current evaluation and management of spondylolysis and spondylolisthesis. *Curr Sports Med Rep* 2003;*2*(1):41–46.

Mellado JM, Lorrosa R, Martin J, Yanguas N, Solanas S, Cozcolluela MR. MDCT of variations and anomalies of the neural arch and its processes: Part I—Pedicles, pars interarticularis, laminae, and spinous process. *AJR Am J Roentgenol* 2011;*197*(1):W104–W113.

History

▶ 22-year-old with proximal tibial pain over several months

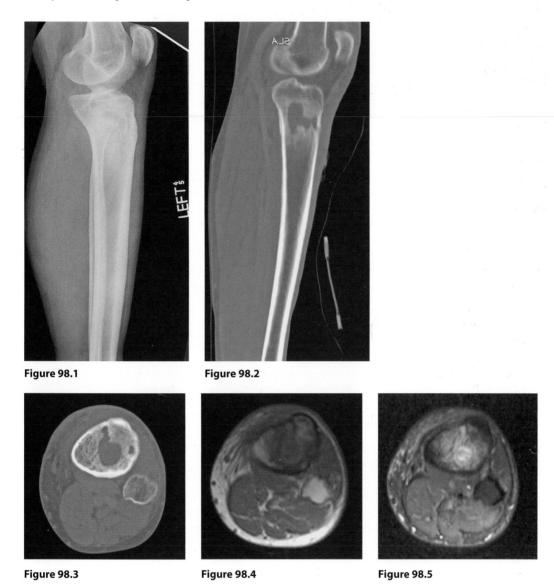

Figure 98.1

Figure 98.2

Figure 98.3

Figure 98.4

Figure 98.5

Case 98 Brodie's abscess (subacute osteomyelitis) of the proximal tibia

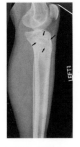 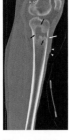 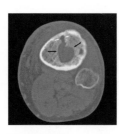 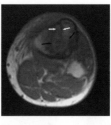 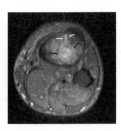

Figure 98.6   **Figure 98.7**   **Figure 98.8**   **Figure 98.9**   **Figure 98.10**

Findings

Radiograph (Fig. 98.6) shows a well-defined, lobular, intramedullary lucency of the proximal tibial metaphysis with moderate surrounding sclerosis (*black arrows*). CT (Figs. 98.7 and 98,8) better demonstrate the lytic lesion and surrounding sclerosis (*black arrows*) and also reveal an associated linear tract extending through the anterior tibial cortex (*white arrows*) consistent with a draining sinus. Adjacent focal anterior soft tissue prominence and skin irregularity are present. Axial MR demonstrates a geographic area of low T1 signal intensity (Fig. 98.9), homogeneous high-signal-intensity STIR fluid with low-signal rim (*black arrows*) (Fig. 98.10) extending to the cortical surface as a sinus tract (*white arrows*), and anterior soft tissue edema.

Differential Diagnosis

Metastasis; lymphoma; eosinophilic granuloma; osteoblastoma or osteoid osteoma; intramedullary infarct or cyst; chondroblastoma (if epiphyseal)

Teaching Points

► Brodie's abscess is a focal, walled-off area of intramedullary infection most common within the metaphysis (femur or tibia) consistent with the subacute or early phase of chronic osteomyelitis (hematogenous type) that may have a draining sinus tract.

► It may occur *de novo* or have a history of prior infection at the same site. *Staphylococcus aureus* is the most common organism. Insidious symptoms leading to late diagnosis include intermittent pain, swelling, and erythema (months to years).While most common in adolescents (2 to 15 years) or young adults, is can be seen up to 61 years of age. Epiphyseal or diaphyseal lesions can occur (Roberts classification system).

► A cloaca, sequestrum, serpentine border, or periosteal reaction may be present on imaging.

► CT is useful to confirm sclerotic margins merging with surrounding bone, suggesting a subacute or chronic process, as well as to localize potential draining sinus. MR further characterizes the collection, intramedullary extent, and potential associated soft tissue abscess or drainage tracts.

Management

Antibiotics are first line of therapy. Incision and drainage is performed if subperiosteal pus is present. Curettage is performed if epiphyseal or metaphyseal lesions communicate with the joint. Care is taken to avoid injuring the growth plate.

Further Readings

Kornaat PR, Camerlinck M, Vanhoenacker FM, De Paeter, Kroon HM. Brodie's abscess revisited. *JBT-BTR* 201;93:81–86.

Poyhia T, Azouz EM. MR imaging evaluation of subacute and chronic bone abscesses in children. *Pediatr Radiol* 2000;*30*(11):763–738.

History

▶ 24-year-old female runner with right hip and groin pain

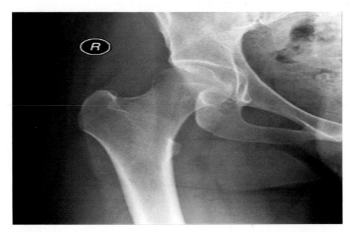

Figure 99.1

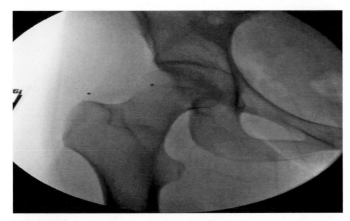

Figure 99.2

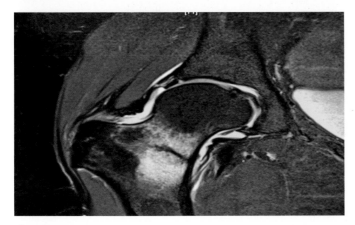

Figure 99.3

Case 99 Stress fracture—femoral neck

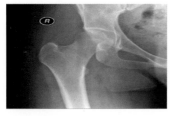

Figure 99.4

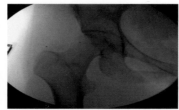

Figure 99.5

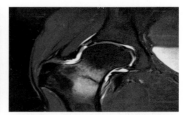

Figure 99.6

Findings

Figure 99.4 (initial radiograph of the right hip) is unremarkable. As there was question of a potential labral tear, an MR arthrogram was performed. Figure 99.5 (arthrographic AP image performed 8 days later) demonstrates linear oblique sclerosis within the inframedial right femoral neck. Figure 99.6 (coronal T2-weighted FS MR arthrogram image) clearly depicts the nondisplaced stress fracture of the inframedial femoral neck, with marked surrounding marrow edema.

Differential Diagnosis

Pathognomonic for femoral neck stress fracture

Teaching Points

▶ Femoral neck stress fractures represent 5% to 10% of all stress fractures and are classified according to location: (1) Inframedial femoral neck (thought to be a compression type of injury) is the most common and can be nondisplaced (nonoperative treatment), as in this case, or may progress to displacement (requiring surgical fixation). (2) Superior femoral neck cortex (high risk of nonunion and complete fracture with potential avascular necrosis—requires surgical pinning).

▶ Given the high complication rate, correct diagnosis is imperative.

▶ Follow-up radiographic images in 7 to 10 days are recommended in healthy adults with hip pain and negative radiographs, particularly in competitive runners, who have a high incidence of stress injuries.

▶ MRI is the gold standard as marrow changes can be seen earlier than radiographic findings in stress reactions or stress fractures. Diffuse edema is characteristic about the linear fracture line. It is also useful for excluding other causes of pain (labral tear) and determining surgical planning. Bone scan in the past proved helpful in initial evaluation but is not specific.

Management

Exclude any underlying pathology that may have led to weakening of the femoral neck if there is no clinical history of running or exertional activity. MR is useful for determining stress reaction versus fracture as well as for excluding any related soft tissue injuries or early complications requiring urgent surgical treatment. Treatment is as noted above for the 2 different locations of stress fractures.

Further Readings

Lee JK, Yao L. Stress fractures: MR imaging. *Radiology* 1988;*169*:217–220.
Manaster BJ. Adult chronic hip pain: Radiographic evaluation. *Radiographics* 2000;*20*:S3–25.

Part V

Internal Derangement of Joints and Soft Tissue Pathology

History

► Runner with lateral knee pain

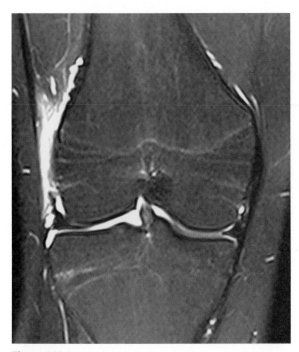

Figure 100.1

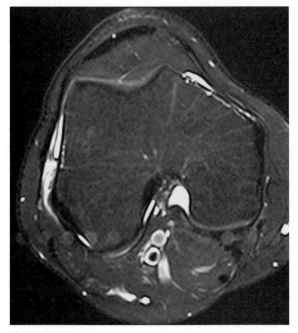

Figure 100.2

Case 100 Iliotibial band syndrome

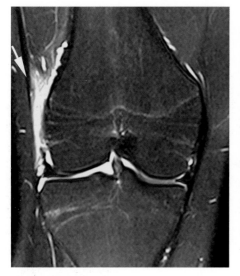

Figure 100.3

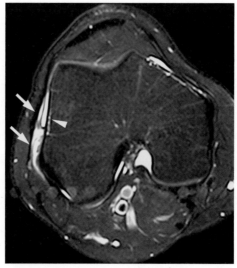

Figure 100.4

Findings

Coronal STIR (Fig. 100.3) and axial fat-saturated T2-weighted (Fig. 100.4) images demonstrate prominent soft tissue fluid and edema between the lateral femoral condyle and iliotibial band (*arrows*). Note the well-circumscribed fluid within the adjacent lateral patellofemoral pouch (*arrowhead*).

Differential Diagnosis

Soft tissue injury from acute trauma (clinical history should differentiate)

Teaching Points

- The iliotibial band syndrome is a common cause of lateral knee pain in athletes and other active individuals involved in activities requiring repetitive flexion/extension of the knee such as running and cycling.
- The associated soft tissue inflammation is thought to result from snapping of the iliotibial band across the lateral femoral condyle, impingement of the intervening fat, development of localized bursitis in this region, or a combination of the three.
- Clinical examination is usually sufficient for diagnosis, but imaging, especially MRI, may be obtained to confirm the diagnosis in questionable cases and rule out other lateral-sided pathology.
- On MRI imaging, fat-saturated T2-weighted images reveal high-signal-intensity soft tissue fluid/edema interposed between the distal iliotibial band and lateral femoral condyle. Joint fluid within the lateral patellofemoral pouch may mimic this condition, but is often recognized by it's sharply marginated appearance within the joint capsule.

Management

Conservative, nonsurgical management (rest, NSAIDs, physical therapy) is usually sufficient, with surgery reserved for only the most recalcitrant cases.

Further Readings

Strauss EJ, Kim S, Calcei JG, Park D. Iliotibial band syndrome: evaluation and management. *J Am Acad Orthop Surg* 2011;*19*:728–736.

History

▶ 15-year-old boy with shoulder pain after injury

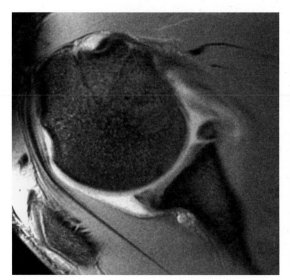

Figure 101.1

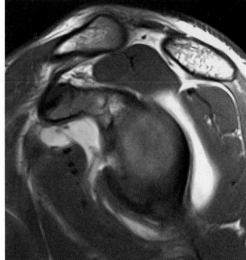

Figure 101.2

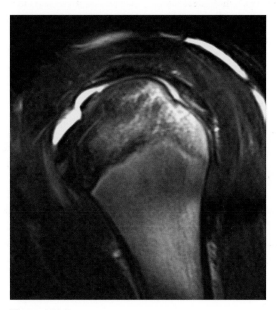

Figure 101.3

Case 101 Sequelae of anterior shoulder dislocation (Hill-Sachs and Bankart lesions)

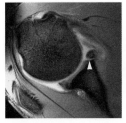

Figure 101.4

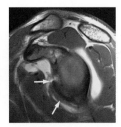

Figure 101.5

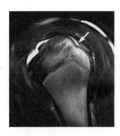

Figure 101.6

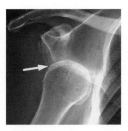

Figure 101.7

Findings

Figure 101.4 (axial gradient echo T2*-weighted image from an MR arthrogram) reveals a tear of the anterior-inferior labrum (cartilaginous Bankart lesion—*arrowhead*). Figure 101.5 (oblique sagittal T1-weighted image) also demonstrates the labral pathology (*arrows*). Figure 101.6 (oblique sagittal fat-saturated T2-weighted image) displays an associated Hill-Sachs impaction fracture along the posterior-superior humeral head and adjacent marrow edema (*arrow*). Figure 101.7 (AP radiograph of the shoulder in a different patient) illustrates the etiology of the Hill-Sachs and Bankart lesions that occur at the point of impact between the humeral head and glenoid in an anterior dislocation (*arrow*).

Differential Diagnosis

None

Teaching Points

▶ Dislocation of the glenohumeral joint is a common injury, and in approximately 90% of cases, the humeral head dislocates in an anterior-inferior direction.

▶ This often results in disruption of the anterior inferior portion of the glenoid labrum (cartilaginous Bankart lesion) or labrum and underlying glenoid rim (osteocartilaginous Bankart) as well as an impaction fracture of the posterior superior aspect of the humeral head (Hill-Sachs lesion).

▶ While these injuries may be evident on radiographs, they are better demonstrated with cross-sectional imaging (CT or MRI).

Management

Relocation of the joint; initial external stabilization; surgical stabilization may be required, especially in patients with recurrent dislocations

Further Readings

Woertler K, Waldt S. MR imaging in sports-related glenohumeral instability. *Eur Radiol* 2006;16:2622–2636.

History

▶ 39-year-old man with sudden onset of shoulder pain and weakness with abnormal electromyographic studies without history of trauma

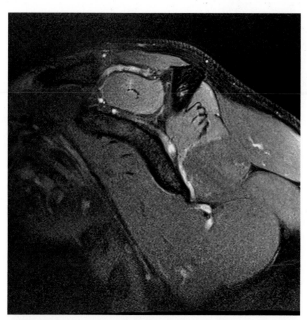

Figure 102.1

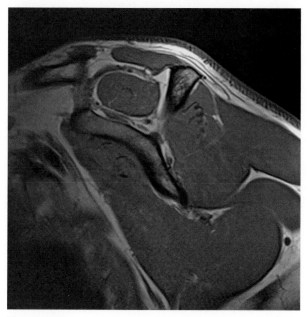

Figure 102.2

Case 102   Parsonage-Turner syndrome (acute idiopathic brachial neuritis)

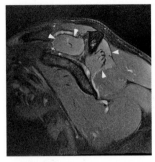

Figure 102.3

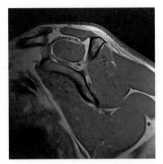

Figure 102.4

Findings

Figures 102.3 and 102.4 (oblique sagittal STIR and T1-weighted MR images) show abnormal increased signal intensity edema isolated to the supraspinatus and infraspinatus muscles (*white arrowheads*) without associated suprascapular or spinoglenoid notch mass or muscle atrophy.

Differential Diagnosis

Pathognonomic

Teaching Points

► Muscle denervation caused by idiopathic brachial neuritis is depicted by increased T2-weighted signal abnormality within the rotator cuff muscles of the shoulder in various combinations, including occasionally the deltoid muscle. The most commonly affected component of the brachial plexus is the suprascapular nerve, which supplies the supraspinatus and infraspinatus muscles. Electromyographic studies are useful for correlation.

► In the acute phase, two thirds of patients will not show any muscle atrophy on MR images (high signal intramuscular fat on T1-weighted images), as in this case. Subacute and chronic phases typically show linear fatty infiltration with decreased muscle bulk with or without associated edema (typically absent in the chronic phase.)

► Need to exclude other causes of nerve compression such as paralabral cyst, rotator cuff tear, ganglion, and in particular masses in particular masses along the course of the suprascapular nerve (suprascapular or spinglenoid notches.)

► Differs from the quadrilateral space syndrome, which has only isolated edema and denervation of the teres minor muscle and, in some cases, deltoid muscles.

Management

Treatment is palliative with analgesics for pain and physical therapy for weakness since this is usually a self-limited condition that uncommonly recurs.

Further Readings

Gaskin C, Helms C. Parsonage-Turner syndrome: MR imaging findings and clinical information of 27 patients. *Radiology* 2006;*240*:501–507.

Scalph R, Wenger D, Frick M, Mandrekar J, Adkins M. MRI Findings of 26 patients with Parsonage Turner syndrome. *AJR Am J Roentgenol* 2007;*189*:39–44.

Yanny S, Toms A. MR Patterns of denervation around the shoulder. *AJR Am J Roentgenol* 2010;*195*:157–163.

History

▶ Right shoulder pain

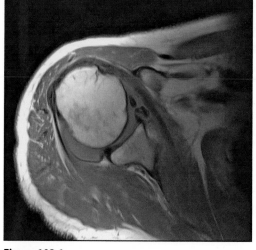

Figure 103.1

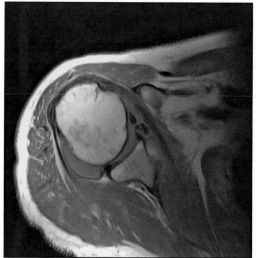

Figure 103.2

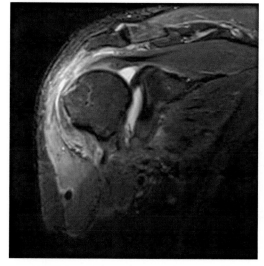

Figure 103.3

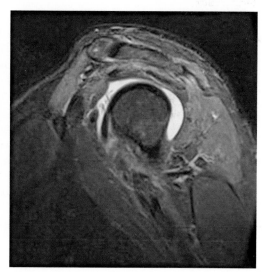

Figure 103.4

Case 103   Medial biceps dislocation (intra-articular)

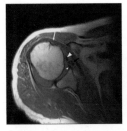

Figure 103.5

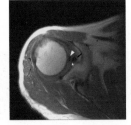

Figure 103.6

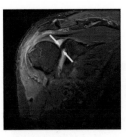

Figure 103.7

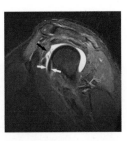

Figure 103.8

Findings

Figures 103.5 and 103.6 (axial T1-weighted MR images) demonstrate an empty biceps groove (*white arrow*) with a round low-signal biceps tendon (*white arrowhead*) within the anterior medial glenohumeral joint space with moderate joint effusion. The anterior labrum (*small white arrowhead*) and middle glenohumeral ligament (*black arrow*) are noted and appear irregular. Figures 103.7 and 103.8 (oblique coronal and oblique sagittal STIR images) confirm a low-signal curvilinear biceps tendon anteromedial to the humeral head (*white arrows*) with absence of the biceps and normal superior glenohumeral ligament within the biceps interval (*black arrow*).

Differential Diagnosis

Loose body; labral tear

Teaching Points

▸ While a low-signal round body within the anteromedial glenohumeral joint could represent a loose body or labral fragment, the absence of the biceps tendon within the groove or in it's normal position within the rotator cuff interval confirms that this is an intra-articular biceps dislocation.

▸ Biceps dislocations are classified as follows:
1. Intra-articular (between the coracohumeral ligament and subscapularis tendon)
   a. Medial displacement of the tendon
   b. Usually in association with disruption of subscapularis tendon and superior glenohumeral ligament and medial coracohumeral ligament complex
   c. Can dislocate anterior to subscapularis but deep to lateral band
2. Extra-articular
   a. Associated with anterolateral supraspinatus tendon tear and lateral coracohumeral ligaments
   b. Tendon subluxes anterior to the lesser tuberosity.
   c. Can have delamination of the deep surface of the subscapularis with biceps tendon subluxed directly into the subscapularis at the site of defect.

▸ Biceps dislocation and entrapment can occur following traumatic dislocations.

Management

Treatment is dependent on type of biceps pulley lesion (from least to most significant): suture repair, debridement with transtendon repair, subscapularis and biceps tendon stabilization, or subscapularis and supraspinatous tendon repair with biceps tenodesis or tenotomy (type 4 lesions).

Further Readings

Morag Y, Jacobson J, Shields G, Rajani R, Jamadar D, Miller B, Hayes C. MR arthrography of rotator interval, long head of the biceps brachii, and biceps pulley of the shoulder. *Radiology* 2005;*235*:21–30.

Stoller D, Wolf E, Li A, Nottage W, Tirman P. The shoulder. In *Magnetic Resonance Imaging in Orthopaedics and Sports Medicine*, 3rd ed., Vol. 2. Baltimore, MD Lippincott Williams and Wilkins: 2007:1131–1146.

History

▶ Shoulder pain without acute injury

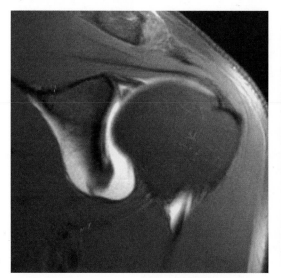

Figure 104.1

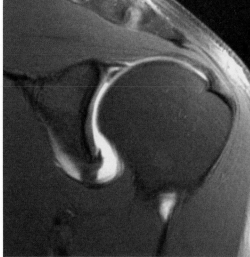

Figure 104.2

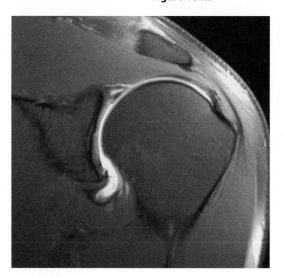

Figure 104.3

Case 104 Superior labral anteroposterior (SLAP) tear

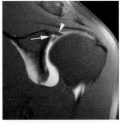 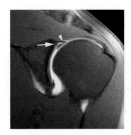 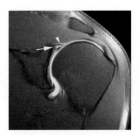 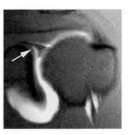

Figure 104.4   **Figure 104.5**   **Figure 104.6**   **Figure 104.7**

Findings

Oblique coronal fat-saturated T1-weighted image at the level of the biceps-labral anchor (*arrowhead* = long head biceps tendon) obtained during an MR arthrogram (Fig. 104.4) reveals abnormal signal intensity within the superior labrum (*arrow*). Figures 104.5 and 104.6 (oblique coronal fat-saturated T1-weighted images just posterior to Fig. 104.4) demonstrate extension of the tear into the posterior superior labrum (*arrows*). Note how the signal intensity is oriented laterally as it extends into the substance of the labrum (*arrowheads*). Figure 104.7 (oblique coronal fat-saturated T1-weighted image obtained during an MR arthrogram in a different patient) shows a sublabral recess. Note how the contrast parallels the superior margin of the glenoid (*arrow*).

Differential Diagnosis

A sublabral recess, a normal variant, may sometimes mimic a SLAP tear but would not have this appearance (see discussion below).

Teaching Points

▶ Tears involving the superior labrum at its attachment to the long head biceps tendon are called superior labral anteroposterior (SLAP) tears.
▶ Numerous types of SLAP tears have been described, with the four original types being (I) fraying of the superior labrum, (II) tear of the superior labrum with stripping of the biceps-labral anchor, (III) longitudinal, bucket-handle type of tear, and (IV) superior labral tear that extends into the proximal biceps tendon.
▶ It may be impossible to differentiate a type II SLAP tear from a sublabral recess, a normal variant in which the superior labrum is loosely attached to the glenoid such that contrast or fluid collects in a small sulcus beneath the labrum.
▶ A helpful differentiating feature, as illustrated in this case, is lateral extension of the abnormal signal intensity into the substance of the labrum in the case of a true tear.

Management

Although conservative treatment (physical therapy, steroid injections) may be attempted, most patients will require arthroscopic repair. In older patients, a biceps tenotomy or tenodesis is often performed.

Further Readings

Modarresi S, Motamedi D, Jude CM. Superior labral anteroposterior lesions of the shoulder: part 1, anatomy and anatomic variants. *AJR Am J Roentgenol* 2011;*197*:596–603.
Modarresi S, Motamedi D, Jude CM. Superior labral anteroposterior lesions of the shoulder: part 2, mechanisms and classification. *AJR Am J Roentgenol* 2011;*197*:604–611.

History

▶ Shoulder pain (two patients, same diagnosis)

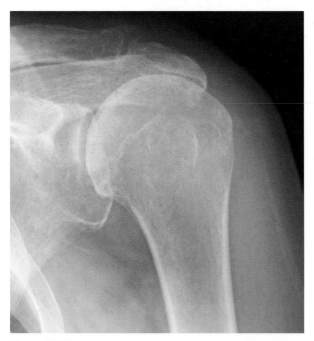

Figure 105.1

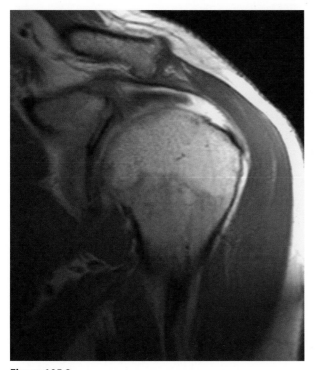

Figure 105.2

Case 105 Full-thickness rotator cuff tear

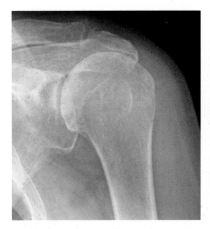

Figure 105.3

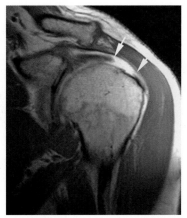

Figure 105.4

Findings

Figure 105.3 (AP radiograph of the left shoulder in external rotation) demonstrates elevation of the humeral head relative to the glenoid with marked narrowing of the humeral acromial distance. Figure 105.4 (oblique coronal T1-weighted image [MR arthrogram] in a different patient) reveals a full-thickness tear of the supraspinatus tendon (*arrows*).

Differential Diagnosis

None

Teaching Points

- ▶ The rotator cuff is made up of the supraspinatus, infraspinatus, teres minor, and subscapularis tendons.
- ▶ Pathology of the rotator cuff tendons is a common cause of shoulder pain and may be the result of traumatic injury or age-related degeneration.
- ▶ Radiographic findings in patients with a full-thickness tear include narrowing of the humeral acromial distance to <6 mm on an AP view or <2 mm on an active abduction view.
- ▶ MR imaging has become the study of choice for evaluation of the rotator cuff given its ability to demonstrate all stages of cuff pathology from tendon degeneration ("tendinosis") to partial-thickness tears to full-thickness tendon disruption.
- ▶ A full-thickness tear is diagnosed when bright fluid is seen extending across the entire affected tendon on T2-weighted images, or as in this case, when gadolinium courses through the tear during an MR arthrogram.
- ▶ Important features of a tear on MR imaging include the size of the tear in two dimensions, the amount of tendon retraction, and any associated fatty atrophy within the cuff muscles.

Management

Conservative measures in cases of suspected cuff pathology include NSAIDs, physical therapy, and corticosteroid injections. Full-thickness tears often require surgical repair.

Further Readings

Buck FM, Grehn H, Hilbe M, Pfirrmann CWA, Manzanell S, Hodler J. Magnetic resonance histologic correlation in rotator cuff tendons. *J Magn Reson Imag* 2010;*32*:165–172.

Moosikasuwan JB, Miller TT, Burke BJ. Rotator cuff tears: clinical radiographic and US findings. *Radiographics* 2005;*25*:1591–1607.

History

▶ Medial ankle pain

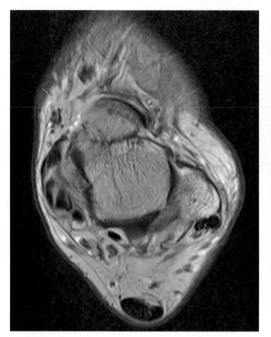

Figure 106.1

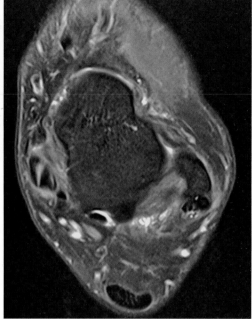

Figure 106.2

Case 106 Split tear of the posterior tibialis tendon (PTT)

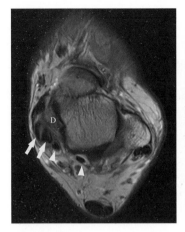 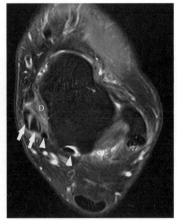

Figure 106.3   **Figure 106.4**

Findings

Figures 106.3 and 106.4 (axial PD and T2 weighted FS MR images) demonstrate abnormal appearance of the medial flexor tendons with two oblong low-signal structures in the expected location of the PTT (*white arrows*) inferomedial to the medial malleolus with linear fluid signal intensity between them. The adjacent Flexor digitorum longus (FDL) and flexor hallucis longus (FHL) tendons appear unremarkable (*white arrowheads*). There is mild sprain of the deep deltoid fibers (D).

Differential Diagnosis

Pathognomonic—the only differential would include potential accessory tendon

Teaching Points

▶ The PTT, FDL, and FHL (three tendons) make up the medial flexor tendon group of the ankle. The normal PTT is typically twice the size of the adjacent FDL and demonstrates homogeneous low signal on all sequences.

▶ The PTT courses inferior medial to the medial malleolus, attaching to the medial pole of the navicular, the plantar aspect of three cuneiforms, as well as the bases of the second to fourth metatarsals, and is the primary longitudinal support for the medial ankle. I most commonly tears where it courses under the medial malleolus secondary to mechanical wear, typically in women over 50 years of age, and in patients with a history of rheumatoid arthritis, steroid use, diabetes and/or renal failure. It may rarely tear acutely in a young athlete.

▶ The PTT is the most commonly torn tendon of the medial ankle and this commonly results in a pes planus deformity that may be evident clinically and on radiographs.

▶ The "4" tendon sign of the medial flexors (rather than the usual 3) on axial MR images is characteristic of the longitudinal split tear of the PTT:

Management

Nonsurgical treatment involves medial longitudinal ligament arch support. Surgical options include débridement, repair, arthrodesis, and side-to-side anastomosis to the flexor digitorum longus tendon.

Further Readings

Ly J. The 4 tendon sign. *Radiology* 2008;247:291–292.
Rosenberg Z, Beltran J, Bencardino J. MR imaging of the ankle and foot. *Radiographics* 2000;*20*:S153–S179.
Schweitzer M, Karasick D. MR imaging of disorders of the posterior tibialis tendon. *AJR Am J Roentgenol* 2000;*175*(3):627–635.

History

▶ 32-year-old woman with lateral foot pain, tenderness, and instability

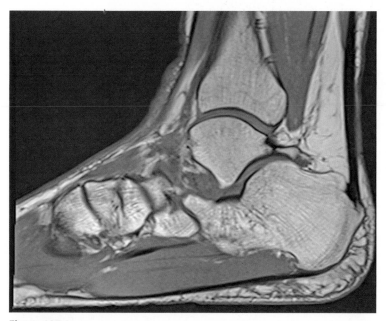

Figure 107.1

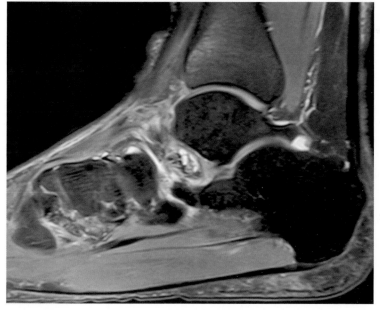

Figure 107.2

Case 107 Sinus tarsi syndrome

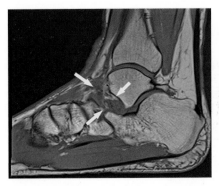
Figure 107.3

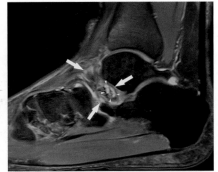
Figure 107.4

Findings

Figures 107.3 (sagittal T1-weighted MR image) and 107.4 (sagittal STIR MR image) demonstrate near-complete replacement of sinus tarsi fat with intermediate T1 signal intensity and abnormal high-signal STIR edema (*white arrows*). A lobulated high-signal-intensity (STIR) fluid collection within the central sinus tarsi is consistent with a small ganglion (*arrowheads*). No associated bone marrow edema, cortical abnormality or fracture present.

Differential Diagnosis

Usually pathognomonic on MR

Teaching Points

▶ Sinus tarsi syndrome was first described by Shear et al. in 1993 and refers to anything that involves, replaces, or invades the region of the sinus tarsi (a fat-, ligament-, and artery-filled space between the talus, calcaneus, and navicular) and results in the following characteristic symptoms:
  – Pain over the lateral foot (should be considered in the differential of lateral ankle pain)
  – Increased tenderness over sinus tarsi area
  – A sense of hindfoot or subtalar instability
  – Pain reproduced by forceful supination of the forefoot
▶ Causes: Trauma (most common) resulting in ligament injury and scar formation; inflammatory arthritis, space occupying mass such as a ganglion or varicosities
▶ Contents of the sinus tarsi include (lateral to medial): inferior extensor retinaculum (lateral, intermediate, and medial roots) (low signal MRI); cervical ligament (low signal MRI); interosseous talocalcaneal ligament (low signal MRI); artery of the tarsal canal
▶ Although MR imaging in these patients may reveal replacement of the normal fat within the sinus tarsi by fluid (dark on T1, bright on T2-weighted images) or scar tissue (dark on both T1 and T2-weighted images, these findings are non-specific and must be correlated with the physical examination as this is ultimately a clinical diagnosis.

Management

Treatment of secondary nerve or vascular structure compression, resection of mass for relief of symptoms, or treatment of inflammatory arthropathy if present. Ganglions can be aspirated or injected with steroid under ultrasound guidance, but they typically recur.

Further Readings

Choudhary S. McNally E. Review of common and unusual causes of lateral ankle pain. *Skeletal Radiol* 2011;40(11):1399–1413.
Mansour R, Jibri Z, Kamath S, Mukherjee K, Ostlere S. Persistent ankle pain following a sprain: a review of imaging. *Emerg Radiol* 2011;18(3):211–225.

History

► Hindfoot pain

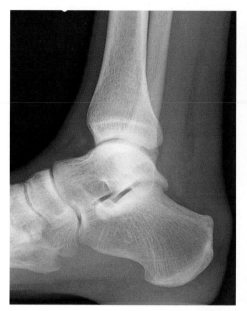

Figure 108.1

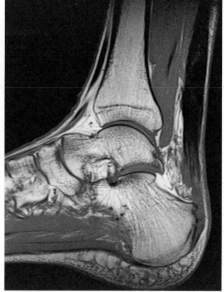

Figure 108.2

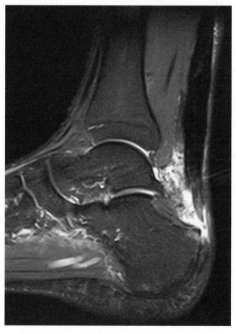

Figure 108.3

Case 108   Chronic Achilles tendinosis and partial tearing ("Haglund's Syndrome")

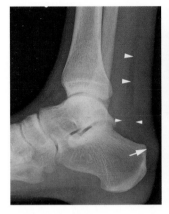 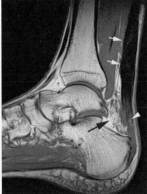 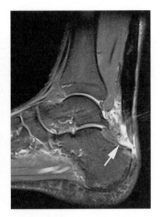

Figure 108.4   **Figure 108.5**   **Figure 108.6**

Findings

Figure 108.4 (lateral radiograph of the hindfoot) shows thickening of the Achilles tendon (*large arrowheads*), focal soft tissue prominence at its calcaneal insertion (*arrow*), and edema infiltrating the pre-Achilles fat pad (*small arrowheads*). Figure 108.5 (sagittal T1-weighted image) reveals marked thickening (*white arrows*) and high-grade partial tearing of the distal Achilles tendon (*arrowhead*) as well as ill-defined edema within the pre-Achilles fat (*black arrow*). Figure 108.6 (sagittal STIR image) better demonstrates fluid distending the pre-Achilles bursa (*arrow*).

Differential Diagnosis

None

Teaching Points

▶ Pathology of the Achilles tendon is usually the result of chronic degeneration that leads to partial or complete tendon tears.

▶ The tearing may occur approximately 5 to 6 cm proximal to its calcaneal insertion in a relatively hypovascular area ("non-insertional") or, as in this case, near its calcaneal attachment ("insertional").

▶ When combined with pre-Achilles bursitis and a palpable "bump" along the dorsum of the heel, this is known as Haglund's syndrome (not to be confused with "Haglund's deformity"—a prominent beaking of the posterior-superior corner of the calcaneus).

▶ Suggestive findings may be evident on radiographs, but MR imaging provides the best depiction of the abnormalities, including the degree of tendon disruption.

Management

Conservative: modified footwear, orthotics, NSAIDs, and potentially image-guided corticosteroid injection into the pre-Achilles bursa. In severe cases, surgical débridement with tendon repair or grafting may be necessary.

Further Readings

Pierre-Jerome C, Moncayo V, Terk MR. MRI of the Achilles tendon: a comprehensive review of the anatomy, biomechanics, and imaging of overuse tendinopathies. *Acta Radiol* 2010;51:438–454.

History

► Throwing athlete with medial elbow pain

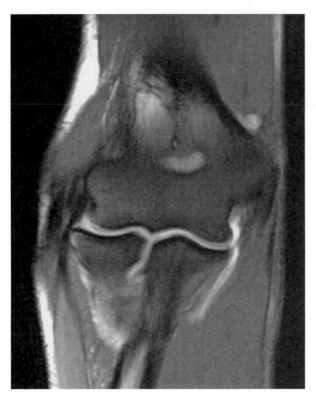

Figure 109.1

Case 109 Tear of the ulnar collateral ligament

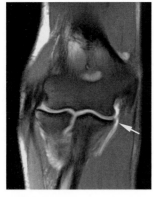
Figure 109.2

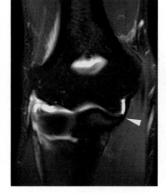
Figure 109.3

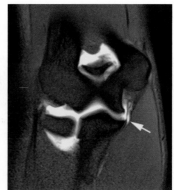
Figure 109.4

Findings

Figure 109.2 (coronal fat-saturated T2-weighted image of the right elbow) reveals disruption of the ulnar collateral ligament at its attachment on the sublime tubercle of the ulna with fluid extending into the adjacent soft tissues (*arrow*). Figure 109.3 (coronal T2-weighted image of the elbow in a different patient) demonstrates a normal attachment of the ligament for comparison (*arrowhead*). Figure 109.4 (coronal T1-weighted image [MR arthrogram] in a college baseball pitcher) demonstrates a partial undersurface tear of the ligament at its distal attachment (*arrow*).

Differential Diagnosis

None

Teaching Points

▶ The ulnar collateral ligament of the elbow extends from the undersurface of the medial humeral epicondyle to the sublime tubercle along the medial aspect of the coronoid process of the ulna.

▶ It is the primary restraint against the valgus force that occurs at the elbow during the throwing motion, and injury can lead to medial elbow pain and instability.

▶ MR imaging can diagnose the degree of tearing and rule out other conditions that may mimic a tear clinically, including pathology of the adjacent common flexor tendon ("medial epicondylitis") or a stress reaction of the medial epicondyle in skeletally immature patients ("Little Leaguer's elbow").

▶ The ligament should demonstrate a tight attachment to the tubercle, and even a small amount of contrast undercutting the ligament indicates a partial tear.

Management

Conservative treatment (typically used in partial tears) includes rest, NSAIDs, and physical therapy. Surgical reconstruction is an option.

Further Readings

Cain, Jr. EL, Dugas JR, Wold RS, Andrews JR. Elbow injuries in throwing athletes: a current concepts review. *Am J Sports Med* 2003;*31*(4):621–635.

History

▸ Right hip pain

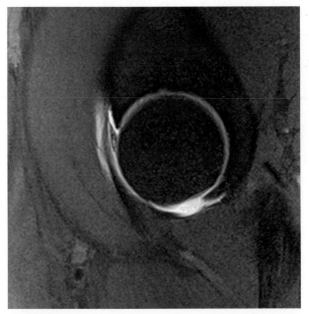

Figure 110.1

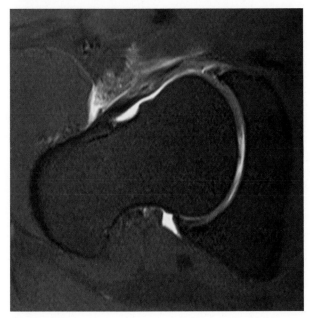

Figure 110.2

Case 110   Anterior superior labral tear

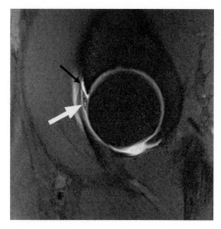

Figure 110.3

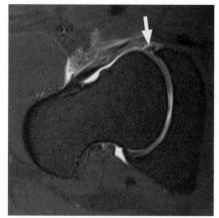

Figure 110.4

Findings

Figures 110.3 and 110.4 (sagittal and axial oblique T1-weighted FS MR arthrogram images) demonstrate complete detachment of the anterior superior labrum at the acetabular junction with high-signal fluid (*black arrow*) extending between the low-signal labral fragment (*white arrow*) and the acetabular rim.

Differential Diagnosis

None

Teaching Points

► Labral evaluation is best performed with an MR arthrogram. The normal labrum should be triangular and demonstrate low signal intensity on all sequences. The labrum is evaluated as a clock face, with anterior superior tears at 10 to 11 o'clock.

► Mildly heterogeneous signal and morphologic changes may be seen with labral degeneration, but frank fluid extending into the labrum indicates a partial or complete tear, with or without detachment. A tear should not be confused with a normal anterior inferior recess (8 o'clock).

► The Czerny classification has traditionally been used, with stage 3A representing complete detachment (as in this case).

► Anterior superior labral tears are most common and best visualized on axial oblique images, followed by sagittal images.

► Associated signs include paralabral cysts, synovial herniation pits, and acetabular cysts.

► There is an increased incidence of labral tears in patients with femoral acetabular impingement syndrome.

Management

Conservative management, with arthroscopic surgical management if symptoms are severe.

Further Readings

Blankenbaker DG, De Smet AA, Keene JS, Fine JP. Classification and localization of acetabular labral tears. *Skeletal Radiol* 2007;*36*(5):391–391.

Ziegert AJ, Blankenbaker DG, De Smet AA, Keene JS, Shinki K, Fine JP. Comparison of standard hip MR arthrographic imaging planes and sequences for detection of arthroscopically proven labral tear. *AJR Am J Roentgenol* 2009;*192*(5):1397–1400.

History

▶ Proximal radial (dorsal lateral) wrist/forearm pain in a tennis player

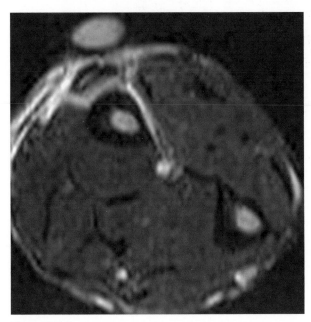

Figure 111.1

Case 111 Intersection syndrome

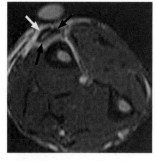

Figure 111.2

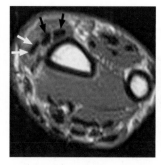

Figure 111.3

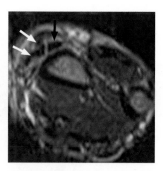

Figure 111.4

Findings

Figure 111.2 (axial STIR MR proximal wrist) demonstrates abnormal dorsal lateral soft tissue edema, with associated tenosynovitis and minimal tendinopathy involving the first extensor compartment (*white arrow*) as it passes over the tendons of the second dorsal compartment (*black arrows*) just proximal to the wrist joint (approximately 5 cm proximal to Lister's tubercle) at the location of dorsolateral pain. Figures 111.3 and 111.4 (axial PD and STIR at the level of the distal forearm) provide better visualization of the tendons of the first (*white arrows*) and second (*black arrows*) extensor compartments and surrounding edema. No tendon tear, fracture, or other bone abnormality is present.

Differential Diagnosis

De Quervain's tenosynovitis; infection; inflammatory tenosynovitis

Teaching Points

▶ Intersection syndrome is characterized by tenosynovitis of BOTH the first and second extensor compartment tendons, with pain and swelling of the first compartment muscle bellies.
▶ The condition is secondary to repetitive overuse with induced friction where the first extensor compartment tendons (abductor pollicis longus and extensor pollicis brevis) cross over the second extensor compartment tendons (extensor carpi radialis and extensor longus brevis) within the distal forearm approximately 5 cm proximal to Lister's tubercle.
▶ Reported associations with sports-related activities including rowing, canoeing, racquet sports, horseback riding, and skiing.
▶ Should be distinguished from De Quervain's tenosynovitis, which involves only the first extensor compartment and produces a positive Finkelstein's test.
▶ Differentiated from infection or inflammatory tenosynovitis by characteristic location and lack of systemic or other findings suggesting arthritis.
▶ An adventitial bursa may occur.

Management

Medical/symptomatic treatment.

Further Readings

Costa C, Morrison W, Carrino J. MR features of intersection syndrome of the forearm. *AJR Am J Roentgenol* 2003;*181*:1245–1243.

Stoller D, Li A, Lichtman D, Brody G. The wrist and hand. In *Magnetic Resonance Imaging in Orthopaedics and Sports Medicine*, 3rd ed., Vol. 2. Baltimore, MD: Lippincott Williams and Wilkins: 2007:1627–1846.

History

► Wrist pain

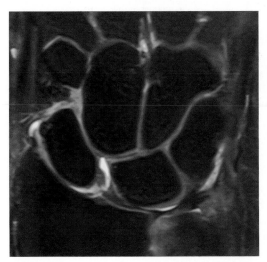

Figure 112.1

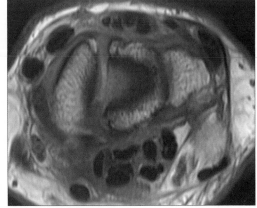

Figure 112.2

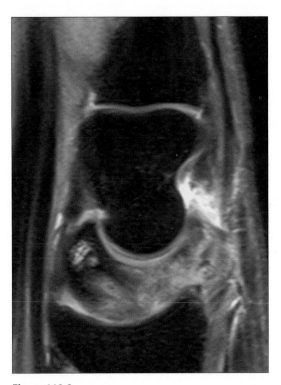

Figure 112.3

Case 112 Scapholunate ligament tear (dorsal and membranous portions)

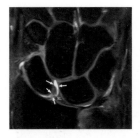
Figure 112.4

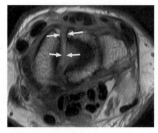
Figure 112.5

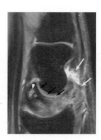
Figure 112.6

Findings

Figure 112.4 (coronal T1-weighted FS MR arthrogram) demonstrates abnormal increased-signal-intensity fluid traversing from the radial carpal joint across the scapholunate ligament (SLL) into the midcarpal joint (*white arrows*). Figure 112.5 (axial T1-weighted MR image) demonstrates minimal abnormal widening of the dorsal SL joint with loss of the normal linear low signal dorsal fibers of the SLL. Taken together, these findings indicate a tear of the membranous and dorsal portions of the SLL (*white arrows*). Associated dorsal edema and extravasated fluid (*white arrows*), dorsal tilt of the lunate articular surface (*black arrows*) characteristic of dorsal intercalated segmental instability (DISI), and subchondral lunate cysts (*arrowhead*) are better seen on the sagittal T2-weighted FS MR sequence (Fig. 112.6).

Differential Diagnosis

Pathognomonic; infection

Teaching Points

▶ The SL ligament has three components (dorsal, middle, and volar), which can be well visualized on axial MR images. The dorsal component is the major stabilizer.

▶ The dorsal and middle components attach to hyaline cartilage or a combination of cartilage and bone, whereas the volar component attaches only to cortical bone.

▶ The normal SL ligament should appear as a triangular, low-signal structure on all sequences without evidence of abnormal high-signal fluid disruption or abnormality in shape. Abnormal extension of fluid across the ligament, best seen on T2-weighted or STIR images (or fat-saturated T1-weighted images in the case of an MR arthrogram) indicates a tear.

▶ The SL ligament can present with degeneration, perforation, partial tear, or complete tear; combinations of the three components can be involved.

▶ SL ligament tears occur preferentially on the side of the scaphoid, as it has a weaker attachment.

▶ Associated findings in SL injuries: widening of the SL joint (>3 mm), proximal scaphoid or lunate edema, subchondral cysts, dorsal intercalated segmental instability (DISI) deformity, dorsal ganglions, synovitis of extrinsic volar ligaments

▶ Can occur with triangular fibrocartilage tears

Management

Conservative treatment with immobilization; surgery in more severe cases.

Further Readings

Schmid M, Schlertler T, Pfirrman C, Saupe M, Manestar M, Wildermuth S, Weishupt D. Interosseous ligament tears of the wrist: comparison of multidetector row CT arthrography and MR imaging. *Radiology* 2005;*185*:1008–1013.

Stoller D, Li A, Lichtman D, Brody G. The wrist and hand. In *Magnetic Resonance Imaging in Orthopaedics and Sports Medicine*, 3rd ed., Vol. 2. Baltimore, MD: Lippincott Williams and Wilkins: 2007:1627–1846.

History

▶ Ulnar-sided wrist pain

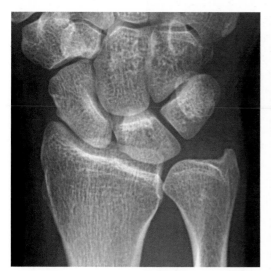

Figure 113.1

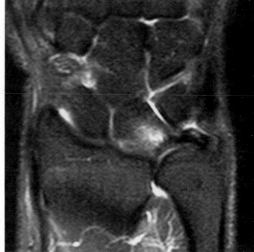

Figure 113.2

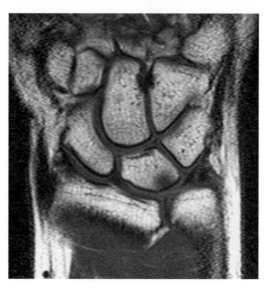

Figure 113.3

Case 113 Ulnolunate abutment syndrome

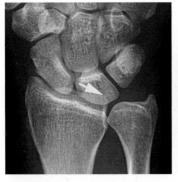

Figure 113.4

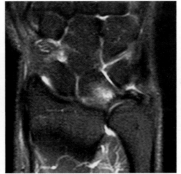

Figure 113.5

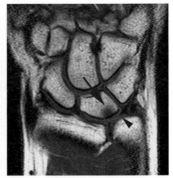

Figure 113.6

Findings

Figure 113.4 (radiograph of the wrist) demonstrates mild positive ulnar variance and subtle subcortical lucencies in the proximal-ulnar aspect of the lunate (*arrow*). Figure 113.5 (coronal STIR image) reveals focal marrow edema within that portion of the lunate, while an adjacent coronal T1-weighted image (Fig. 113.6) shows the edema (*arrow*) as well as a tear of the triangular fibrocartilage (*arrowhead* indicates the ulnar margin of the tear).

Differential Diagnosis

None

Teaching Points

▶ Positive ulnar variance predisposes to mechanical impaction of the ulna against the adjacent lunate or triquetrum, potentially resulting in ulnar-sided wrist pain.

▶ A relatively elongated ulna may represent a congenital variant or may be secondary foreshortening of the distal radius due to a prior impacted fracture or growth plate injury.

▶ The lunate is most frequently involved, and a common associated finding is tearing of the intervening triangular fibrocartilage.

▶ Radiographic findings include positive ulnar variance and subcortical lucencies or sclerosis in the head of the ulna or proximal-ulnar aspect of the lunate.

▶ MR imaging demonstrates subchondral marrow edema at the sites of impaction prior to development of radiographic findings, and may also reveal an associated triangular fibrocartilage tear or chondral loss along the affected articular surfaces.

Management

Conservative treatment includes immobilization, NSAIDs, and corticosteroid injections. Surgical options include ulnar shortening procedures or removal of a portion of the ulnar head ("wafer" procedure).

Further Readings

Sachar K. Ulnar-sided wrist pain: evaluation and treatment of triangular fibrocartilage complex tears, ulnocarpal impaction syndrome, and lunotriquetral ligament tears. *J Hand Surg Am* 2008;*33*:1669–1679.

History

▶ Young gymnast with elbow pain

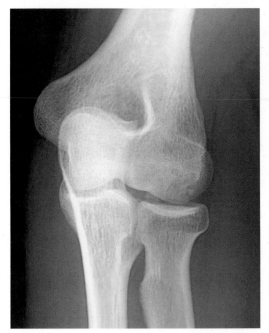

Figure 114.1

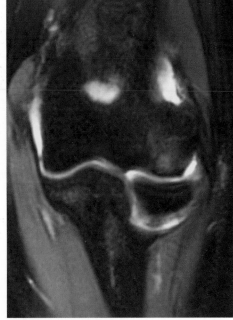

Figure 114.2

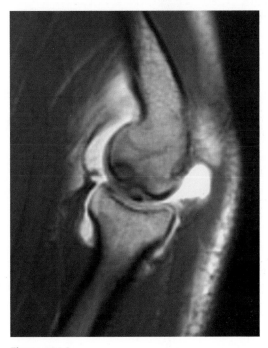

Figure 114.3

Case 114 Osteochondral lesion of the capitellum ("osteochondritis dissecans")

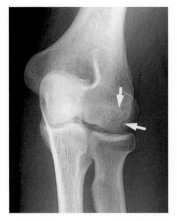

Figure 114.4

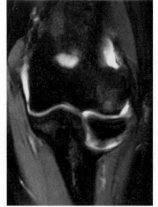

Figure 114.5

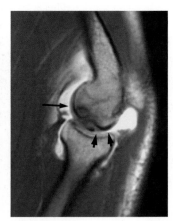

Figure 114.6

Findings

Figure 114.4 (frontal radiograph of the elbow) demonstrates an irregular focus of subchondral lucency in the capitellum (*arrows*). Figure 114.5 (coronal fat-saturated T2-weighted image [MR arthrogram]) reveals abnormal increased signal within the marrow of the capitellum. Figure 114.6 (sagittal T1-weighted image) shows heterogeneous subchondral signal in that portion of the capitellum without evidence of contrast extending into the bone ("stable fragment"). Note the intact cartilage over the ventral portion of the capitellum (*long arrow*) and focal cartilage thinning along its distal aspect (*short arrows*).

Differential Diagnosis

Subchondral capitellar contusion related to acute trauma

Teaching Points

► Repetitive trauma to the capitellum may result in an area of subchondral injury and chronic elbow pain.
► Formerly known as osteochondritis dissecans, it has more recently been called an osteochondral lesion, likely to emphasize its presumptive relationship to chronic trauma. Similar entities are found in the knee (inner, non-weightbearing portion of the medial femoral condyle) and ankle (talar dome).
► Capitellar involvement is most commonly seen in throwers, in whom it is thought to result from chronic impaction forces that develop secondary to progressive failure of the ulnar collateral ligament.
► The primary role of MR imaging is to try to ascertain whether the commonly associated subchondral fragment is stable or unstable. An unstable fragment is diagnosed when fluid or contrast (in the case of an MR or CT arthrogram) insinuates between the fragment and underlying bone; this is the primary imaging finding seen with an unstable fragment. The status of the overlying articular cartilage should also be assessed.

Management

Arthroscopic removal of an unstable fragment versus fixation of the fragment versus osteochondral plug transfer procedure

Further Readings

Kijowski R, DeSmet AA. MRI findings of osteochondritis dissecans of the capitellum with surgical correlation. *AJR Am J Roentgenol* 2005;*185*:1453–1459.

History

▸ Felt pop in elbow with sudden onset of pain

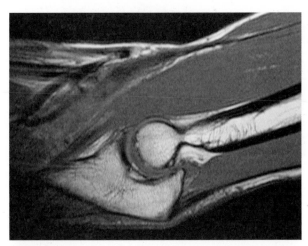

Figure 115.1

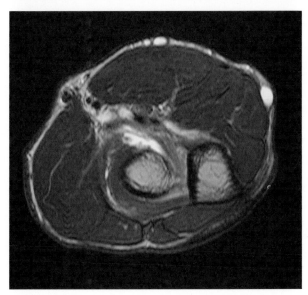

Figure 115.2

Case 115 Complete tear of the distal biceps tendon

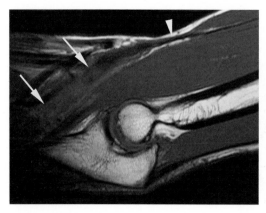

Figure 115.3

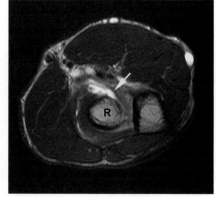

Figure 115.4

Findings

Figure 115.3 (sagittal T1-weighted image) reveals a thickened and ill-defined distal biceps tendon (*arrows*). Note the more normal-appearing proximal portion of the tendon (*arrowhead*). Figure 115.4 (axial fat-saturated T2-weighted image) reveals a complete tear of the distal biceps with absence of the tendon at its attachment site on the radial tuberosity (*arrow*; R = radius).

Differential Diagnosis

None

Teaching Points

▶ The distal biceps tendon courses from the upper arm to insert on the radial tuberosity just distal to the elbow joint. It assists with both flexion and supination of the forearm.

▶ The spectrum of tendon pathology ranges from tendinosis (chronic degeneration) to a complete tear.

▶ Classically, the patient will describe feeling a "pop" or sudden pain within the elbow, and may present with a palpable mass in the distal upper arm due to proximal migration of the torn tendon.

▶ Imaging plays an important role in differentiating partial from complete tears, especially when the tendon is not significantly retracted (as in this case). US may be used for evaluating the biceps tendon, but it can be very challenging to accurately assess its distal fibers with this technique. MRI is able to provide a better overall assessment of the tendon, but the axial scans must extend completely through the radial tuberosity for accurate diagnosis.

Management

Tendinosis and some partial tears are treated conservatively, but more extensive partial and complete tears will be addressed surgically.

Further Readings

Blease S, Stoller S, Safran M, Li A, Fritz R. Chapter 10: The elbow. In Stoller DW, ed. *Magnetic Resonance Imaging in Orthopaedics and Sports Medicine,* 3rd ed. Philadelphia: Lippincott Williams & Wilkins, 2006.

Quach T, Jazayeri R, Sherman OH, Rosen JE. Distal biceps tendon injuries: current treatment options. *Bull NYU Hosp Joint Dis* 2012;68:103–111.

Williams BD, Schweitzer ME, Weishaupt D, et al. Partial tears of the distal biceps tendon: MR appearance and associated clinical findings. *Skeletal Radiol* 2001;30:560–564.

History

▶ Medial elbow pain and paresthesias

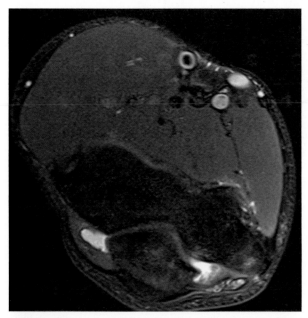

Figure 116.1

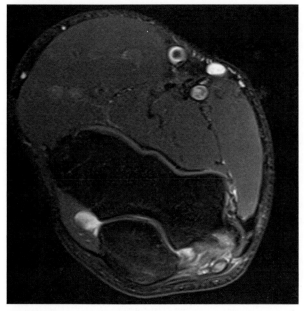

Figure 116.2

Case 116   Cubital tunnel syndrome

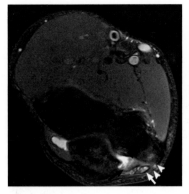

Figure 116.3

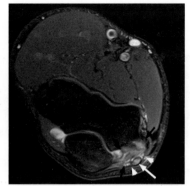

Figure 116.4

Findings

Figures 116.3 and 116.4: Axial STIR MR images of the elbow depict medial subluxation of a minimally enlarged ulnar nerve which demonstrates increased signal intensity (*white arrows*) along with bowing and partial disruption of the cubital tunnel retinaculum (*white arrowheads*). There is associated soft tissue edema within the posteromedial cubital tunnel (*black arrows*). Mild increased-signal bone marrow edema is present within the olecranon and medial epicondyle of the humerus (*black arrowheads*).

Differential Diagnosis

Cubital tunnel mass; medial epicondylitis; infection

Teaching Points

- ▶ Cubital tunnel syndrome is the second most common peripheral neuropathy of the upper extremity and is due to compression of the ulnar nerve behind the medial epicondyle.
- ▶ Enlargement of the ulnar nerve and intraneural T2 hyperintensity are characteristic.
- ▶ Patients present with medial elbow pain that increases on flexion with or without muscle weakness.
- ▶ Classified into physiologic and compression syndromes; causes include pathologic compression by soft tissue mass or accessory anconeus muscle, thickened retinaculum, repetitive microtrauma ("cocking motion" in pitchers), sleep palsy (prolonged flexion/external rotation), humeral fracture, synovitis, infection, and ulnar nerve subluxation due to congenital laxity of fibrous tissue or tear of the retinaculum with associated swelling
- ▶ Ulnar subluxation occurs in 16% of individuals and may be asymptomatic.
- ▶ Medial epicondylitis may be seen in association with this entity in cases of trauma, overuse, or repetitive subluxation of the ulnar nerve.
- ▶ Selective denervation edema and atrophy of the flexor carpi ulnaris and flexor digitorum profundus muscles can occur in ulnar neuropathy and is best identified on axial MR images.

Management

Conservative management is most common: NSAIDS, immobilization or elbow pad placement or splint for up to 3 months. Lidocaine or corticosteroid injections may help. Surgical therapy only if conservative therapy fails: *in situ* decompression, *in situ* decompression with medial epicondylectomy or anterior transposition.

Further Readings

Andreisek G, Crook D, Burg D, Marincek B, Weishaupt D. Peripheral neuropathies of the median, radial and ulnar nerves: MR imaging features. *Radiographics* 2006;*26*:1267–1287.

Blease S, Stoller S, Safran M, Li A, Fritz R. Chapter 10: The elbow. In *Magnetic Resonance Imaging in Orthopaedics and Sports Medicine*, 3rd ed., Vol. 2. Baltimore, MD: Lippincott Williams and Wilkins: 2007:1463–1626.

History

▶ Foot drop

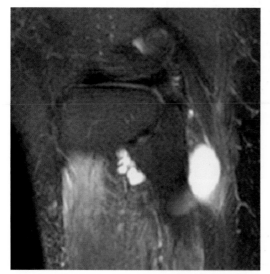

Figure 117.1

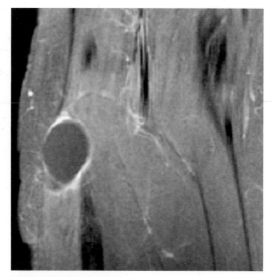

Figure 117.2

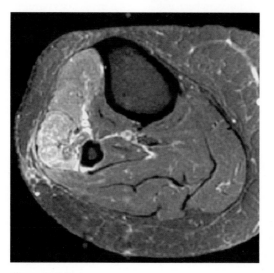

Figure 117.3

Case 117   Ganglion cyst compressing common peroneal nerve, resulting in denervation of the muscles of the anterior and lateral compartments of the calf

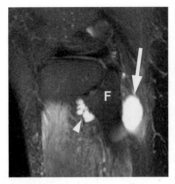
Figure 117.4

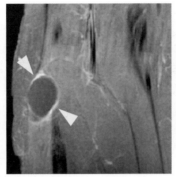
Figure 117.5

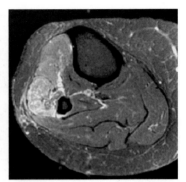
Figure 117.6

Findings

Figure 117.4 (sagittal STIR image at the level of the proximal tibiofibular joint) demonstrates an ovoid, high-signal-intensity mass (*arrow*) posterior to the proximal fibula (*F*). A small cluster of similar-appearing lesions is seen anterior to the fibula as well (*arrowhead*). Figure 117.5 (coronal contrast-enhanced, fat-saturated T1-weighted image) shows only thin peripheral enhancement in the mass (*arrowheads*), compatible with a cyst. Figure 117.6 (axial fat-saturated T2-weighted image at the level of the proximal calf) demonstrates diffuse, edema-like signal intensity within the anterior compartment and peroneal muscles, compatible with acute to subacute denervation.

Differential Diagnosis

None. For muscle "edema" alone, the differential is extensive and includes muscle injury, ischemia, radiation change, as well as inflammatory or primary muscle disorders.

Teaching Points

▶ Injury to a nerve will result in pathologic changes in the muscles innervated by that nerve, which are reflected in their MR imaging appearance.

▶ In the acute to subacute phases, increased fluid content within the affected muscles is manifest as increased, edema-like signal intensity on fluid-sensitive T2-weighted images obtained with fat saturation. The changes are reversible in these stages if the muscle is reinnervated.

▶ After several months, fatty replacement of the muscle develops and is seen best on T1-weighted images as areas of abnormal increased intramuscular signal. This represents irreversible muscle atrophy.

▶ Between these two stages, both edema-like signal and fatty changes are seen on MR images.

Management

Surgical management (excision of a compressing mass or repair of a damaged nerve) may be necessary.

Further Readings

Kamath S, Venkatanarasimha N, Hughes PM. MRI appearance of muscle denervation. *Skeletal Radiol* 2008;37:397–404.

History

▸ 14-year-old female soccer player who noticed a mass in her right thigh

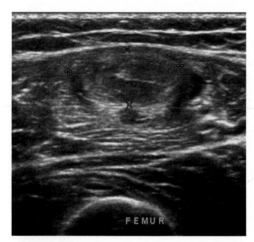

Figure 118.1

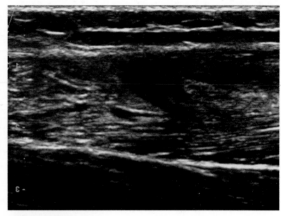

Figure 118.2

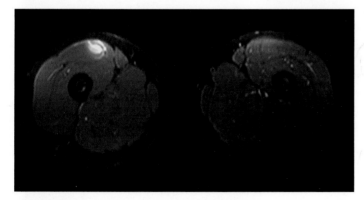

Figure 118.3

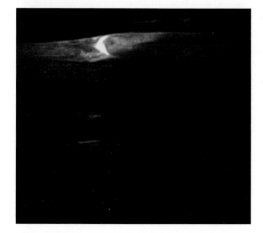

Figure 118.4

Case 118　Partial tear, rectus femoris muscle

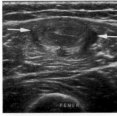
Figure 118.5

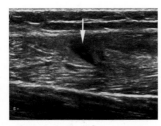
Figure 118.6

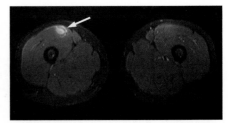
Figure 118.7

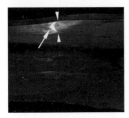
Figure 118.8

Findings

Figure 118.5 (transverse ultrasound image of the anterior mid-thigh at the site of the patient's "mass") reveals a focal ovoid area of heterogeneous echotexture within the rectus femoris muscle (*arrows*). Figure 118.6 (longitudinal scan at the same level) demonstrates a hypoechoic defect indicating a partial tear of the muscle (*arrow*). Corresponding fat-saturated T2-weighted axial (Fig. 118.7) and sagittal (Fig. 118.8) scans confirm the partial rectus femoris tear (*arrows*) with surrounding edema/hemorrhage. The "mass" on the initial transverse sonogram is shown to represent the torn, proximally retracted muscle fibers (*arrowheads* in Fig. 118.8).

Differential Diagnosis

None

Teaching Points

▶ Muscle injuries are most common in those that cross two joints, such as the quadriceps, hamstrings, and gastrocnemius muscles.
▶ These injuries most typically involve the myotendinous junction and are classically separated into three grades:
　– *Grade I* = strain (interstitial injury without macroscopic fiber disruption)
　▪ US: normal or subtle hyperechoic areas within the muscle; perifascial fluid
　▪ MRI: feathery interstitial high-signal edema on T2-weighted images
　– *Grade II* = partial tear
　▪ US/MRI: discontinuity of muscle fibers, often with a focal fluid collection
　– *Grade III* = complete tear
　▪ US/MRI: complete disruption of muscle fibers, often with a hypoechoic (US)/hyperintense (MRI T2-weighted) hematoma between the torn margins

Management

Conservative measures with grades 1 and 2 injuries. Surgical repair may be necessary with complete ruptures to avoid tear extension, scar formation, and/or muscle atrophy.

Further Readings

Lee JC, Healy J. Sonography of lower limb muscle injury. *AJR Am J Roentgenol* 2004;*182*:341–351.

History

▶ 19-year-old male with knee pain post trauma

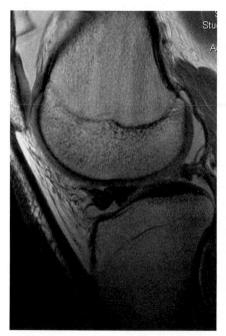

Figure 119.1

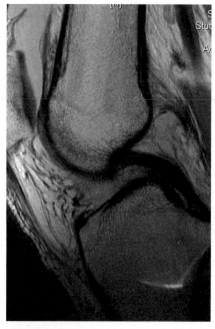

Figure 119.2

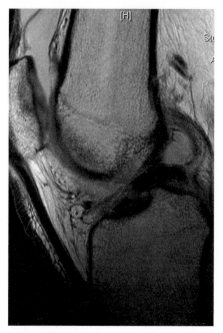

Figure 119.3

Case 119 Bucket-handle tear

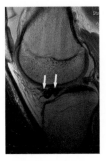 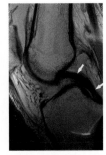 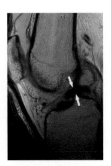

Figure 119.4   **Figure 119.5**   **Figure 119.6**

Findings

Figure 119.4 (sagittal PD MR image) demonstrates loss of the normal bowtie appearance of the lateral meniscus with two low-signal triangular structures in the expected region of its anterior horn ("double delta sign") (*white arrows*) along with a small posterior horn. Figure 119.5 (sagittal PD MR image) confirms that the posterior cruciate ligament (PCL) is intact (*white arrows*); however, there is a second inferiorly placed intercondylar curvilinear low-signal meniscal fragment (*white arrows*) that parallels the PCL, identified on Fig. 119.6 (sagittal PD MR image).

Differential Diagnosis

In this case there really is no differential diagnosis; however, one could potentially consider loose body; torn ligament; prominent transverse meniscal ligaments; prominent meniscofemoral ligament (Humphrey).

Teaching Points

► A bucket-handle tear is a displaced longitudinal tear of the meniscus. The separated central fragment is the bucket handle and the remaining peripheral meniscus is the bucket.
► It is common in young patients post trauma.
► Medial bucket handle tears are three times more common than lateral tears.
► Lateral meniscal tears depict more anterior displacement of posterior horn tissue than medial tears.
► Bucket-handle tears are characterized by three MR signs, all best visualized on sagittal MR images:
   1. The "double delta sign" refers to two triangular low-signal structures within the anterior portion of the meniscus (the flipped inner meniscal fragment is posterior to the anterior horn of the donor site).
   2. The "double PCL sign" refers to the centrally displaced curvilinear low-signal bucket-handle fragment in the intercondylar notch paralleling the PCL anteriorly and is more commonly identified with medial bucket handle tears.
   3. The "absent bowtie sign" refers to loss of the normal sagittal bowtie appearance of the meniscus on peripheral images due to loss of the width of the meniscus caused by the bucket-handle tear.
► Bucket-handle tears have a high association with anterior cruciate ligament injuries.
► Double bucket-handle tears (both medial and lateral tears) can occur, demonstrating two fragments rather than a single fragment within the intercondylar notch on coronal MR images.

Management

Surgical repair of any bucket handle tear if the tear is in or near the vascular periphery and the fragment is not morphologically deformed.

Further Readings

Dorsay TA, Helms CA. Bucket-handle meniscal tears of the knee: sensitivity and specificity of MR signs. *Skeletal Radiol* 2003;32(5):266–273.
Vande Berg B, Malghem J, Poilvache P, Maldague B, Lecouvet F. Meniscal tears with fragments displaced in notch and recesses of knee: MR imaging with arthroscopic correlation. *Radiology* 2005;234:842–850.

History

▶ Medial knee pain after injury

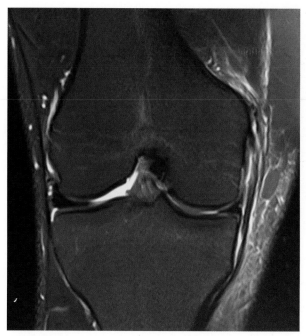

Figure 120.1

Case 120 Partial tear of the medial collateral ligament

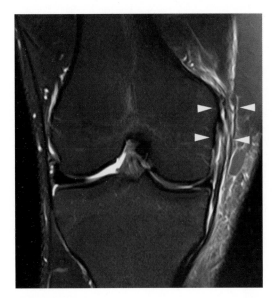

Figure 120.2

Findings

Figure 120.2 (coronal fat-saturated T2-weighted image) demonstrates prominent fluid and edema involving the medial collateral ligament (MCL) as well as partial tearing of its proximal fibers (*arrowheads*).

Differential Diagnosis

None

Teaching Points

- ▶ The MCL is the primary restraint to valgus force at the knee and is commonly injured in a variety of sports.
- ▶ The ligament is composed of a superficial component that extends from the medial femoral condyle to the proximal tibial metaphysis approximately 5 to 7 cm distal to the joint line. The fibers of the deep component attach directly to the medial meniscus and extend to the adjacent femoral condyle and tibial plateau.
- ▶ MCL injuries are clinically graded as a sprain (Grade 1—tenderness with no instability), partial tear (Grade 2—tenderness and laxity with a firm endpoint), and complete tear (Grade 3—laxity with no endpoint).
- ▶ The MCL is best demonstrated on coronal MR images and normally demonstrates low signal intensity on all sequences.
- ▶ A sprain is diagnosed when fluid/edema is seen adjacent to an otherwise intact ligament. Partial disruption of the deep or superficial fibers, as in this case, constitutes a partial tear, and a complete tear is diagnosed when there is complete disruption without any fibers in continuity.

Management

Grades 1 and 2 injuries are often treated conservatively with a brace. A grade 3 tear may be treated conservatively but may require surgery, especially if it is part of a multiligamentous injury.

Further Readings

Kurzweil PR, Kelley ST. Physical examination and imaging of the medial collateral ligament and posteromedial corner of the knee. *Sports Med Arthosc Rev* 2006;14:67–73.

Part VI

Metabolic, Hematologic, and Marrow Disorders

History

▶ 46-year-old woman with knee pain. No history of trauma.

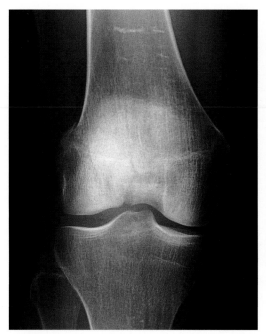

Figure 121.1

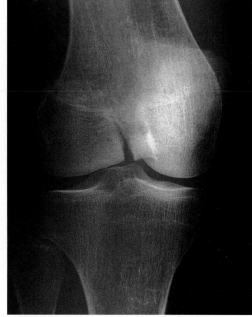

Figure 121.2

Case 121 Severe, diffuse osteopenia with an associated insufficiency fracture of the lateral femoral condyle. Patient had a history of anorexia nervosa

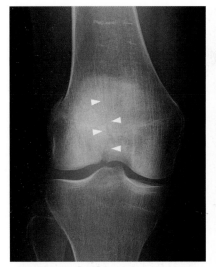

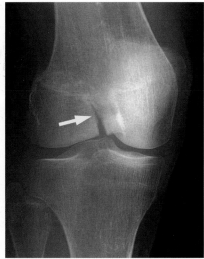

Figure 121.3

Figure 121.4

Findings

AP (Fig. 121.3) radiograph reveals severe osteopenia of the bones of the knee with a subtle vertically oriented fracture line (*arrowheads*) that is better demonstrated on an oblique view (Figure 121.4, *arrow*). Note the prominent trabecular bars in the distal femur as well as the thin, sharply defined cortices.

Differential Diagnosis

Diffuse osteopenia: osteoporosis, hyperparathyroidism, osteomalacia, tumor (usually multiple myeloma).

For true osteoporosis (acronym: AMEDICAL): **A**ge-related bone loss (affects men and women); **M**edications (steroids, heparin, Dilantin, others); **E**ndocrine (menopause, amenorrhea, Chusing's disease, hypogonadism); **D**iet (poor calcium intake, anorexia and other eating disorders); **C**ongential (osteogenesis imperfect); **A**nemia (sickle cell, thalassemia); **L**iver disease.

Teaching Points

▶ Radiographic features suggesting osteoporosis as the etiology of diffuse osteopenia include the following:
  ▪ Thin but very sharply defined cortices and trabeculae
  ▪ Prominent trabecular bars (as seen in the distal femur of this patient)
▶ Insufficiency fractures result from normal stresses applied to abnormal bone, whereas fatigue fractures are related to excessive forces applied to normal bone.

Management

Acute: treatment of any insufficiency fractures. Chronic: medical treatment with calcium supplementation and possibly bone-forming agents.

Further Readings

Bauer JS, Link TM. Advances in osteoporosis imaging. *Eur J Radiol* 2009;71:440–449.
Golden NH. Osteopenia and osteoporosis in anorexia nervosa *Adolesc Med.* 2003;14:97–108.

History

▶ Child with ankle pain

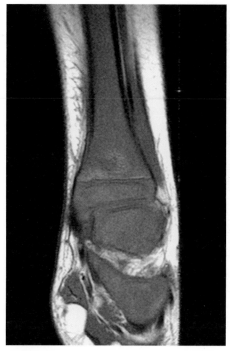

Figure 122.1

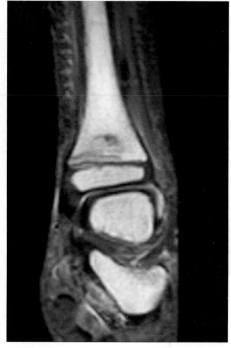

Figure 122.2

Case 122 Leukemia

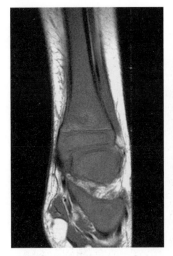

Figure 122.3

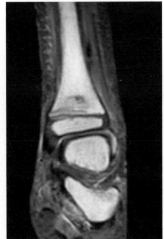

Figure 122.4

Findings

Figure 122.3 (coronal T1-weighted image of the left ankle) reveals diffusely decreased signal intensity throughout the marrow of the distal tibia and bones of the hindfoot that demonstrates markedly increased signal intensity on a corresponding coronal STIR image (Fig. 122.4). (The poorly marginated area of ill-defined signal within the marrow of the distal tibial metaphysis in Fig. 122.4 is related to a biopsy at that site.)

Differential Diagnosis

Severe anemia; diffuse metastatic disease. Other marrow-replacing processes such as osteomyelitis or Langerhans cell histiocytosis would be very unlikely given the diffuse, polyostotic involvement.

Teaching Points

- ▶ Leukemia is the most common neoplasm of childhood.
- ▶ Radiographic findings are common at the time of presentation and include lucent metaphyseal bands, periosteal reaction, osteopenia, osteosclerosis, or a mixed lytic/sclerotic appearance. Radiographs in this case were normal (not shown).
- ▶ MR imaging is very sensitive for detecting a diffuse marrow-replacing process such as leukemia, and may detect the disease even earlier than bone marrow aspiration.
- ▶ Even in a young child, some yellow (fatty) marrow will be evident in an extremity and can be identified by its increased signal intensity on T1-weighted images, paralleling that of the subcutaneous fat.
- ▶ Diffuse or focal signal intensity equal to or lower than that of adjacent muscle on T1-weighted images, as in this case, is worrisome for neoplasm and should prompt further investigation.

Management

Chemotherapy and possible bone marrow transplantation

Further Readings

Kato M, Katsuyoshi K, Kikuchi A, et al. Case series of pediatric acute leukemia without a peripheral blood abnormality, detected by magnetic resonance imaging. *Int J Hematol* 2011;*93*:787–790.

Sinigaglia R, Gigante C, Bisinella G, Varotto S, Zanesco L, Turra S. Musculoskeletal manifestations in pediatric acute leukemia. *J Pediatr Orthop* 2008;*28*:20–28.

History

▶ 35-year-old woman with knee pain and history of underlying systemic disorder

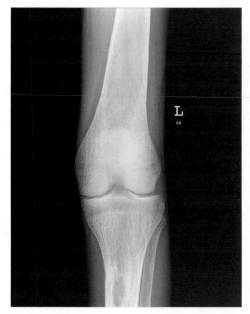

Figure 123.1

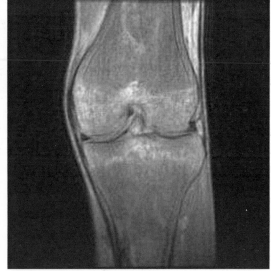

Figure 123.2

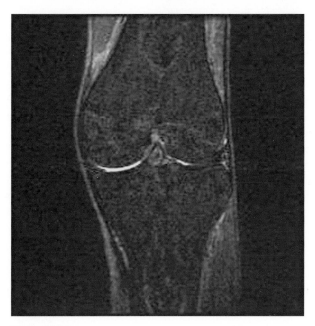

Figure 123.3

Case 123   Sickle cell anemia

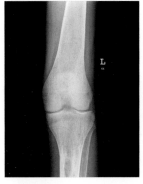

Figure 123.4

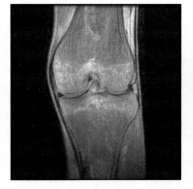

Figure 123.5

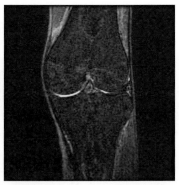

Figure 123.6

Findings

Figure 123.4 (AP radiograph of the knee) demonstrates increased patchy sclerosis of the ossific structures and loss of the normal tubulation of the distal femur and proximal tibia. Figures 123.5 and 123.6 (coronal T1-weighted and STIR images of the knee) depict abnormal signal intensity throughout the marrow of the distal femur and proximal tibia (low signal intensity on both sequences). Pertinent negatives include no soft tissue collection or periosteal reaction or fracture.

Differential Diagnosis

Metastatic disease; myeloma; Gaucher's disease; glycogen storage disease; lymphoma

Teaching Points

▶ Sickle cell anemia is an autosomal recessive condition characterized by the defective hemoglobin S (HbS). Deoxygenation of HbS-containing red blood cells (RBCs) causes aggregation of Hb molecule, distortion of the RBC and resulting microcirculation, ischemia, infarction, and anemia from the rapid removal of abnormal RBCs.

▶ The need for increased production of RBCs in sickle cell patients stops the normal conversion of red to yellow marrow—hence persistent red marrow with resulting persistent low marrow signal changes, as in this patient.

▶ Bone marrow expansion with cortical thinning (typically skull and spine) gives rise to an increased risk of fractures.

▶ Painful bone crises are common with marrow infarction leading to osteolysis initially followed later by sclerosis giving rise to a mottled appearance and remodeling of the bones. Premature fusion of growth plates can also occur.

▶ "Fish–mouth" or "H-shaped" appearance of vertebral bodies (increased endplate compressions), osteopenia, fractures, osteomyelitis (typical organism is Salmonella) and extramedullary hematopoiesis are other complications.

Management

MR imaging is the best modality for confirming the marrow abnormalities in this disease although CT and radionuclide scanning may also be useful for excluding other complications such as osteomyelitis or fracture.

Further Readings

Ejindu VC, Hine AL, Mashayekhi M, Shorvon PJ, Misra RR. Musculoskeletal manifestations of sickle cell disease. *Radiographics* 2007;*27*:1005–1021.

Lonergan GJ, Cline DB, Abbondanzo SL. Sickle cell anemia. *Radiographics* 2001;*21*:971–994.

History

▶ Young woman with recent onset of bilateral hip pain

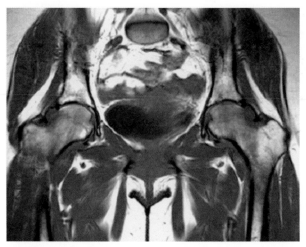

Figure 124.1

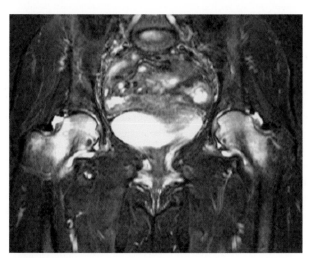

Figure 124.2

Case 124 Transient bone marrow edema syndrome of the hips

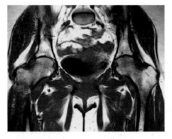
Figure 124.3

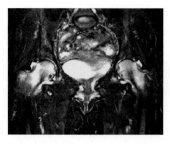
Figure 124.4

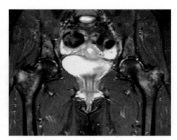
Figure 124.5

Findings

Coronal T1-weighted (Fig. 124.3) and STIR (Fig. 124.4) images of the pelvis demonstrate diffuse, edema-like signal within both proximal femurs as well as small bilateral hip effusions. Figure 124.5 (coronal STIR image of the pelvis obtained 10 weeks later) reveals a significant decrease in the marrow abnormalities. The patient reported an interval improvement in symptoms at this time as well.

Differential Diagnosis

Avascular necrosis, although this diagnosis is typically reserved for cases demonstrating irregular, often flame-shaped areas of abnormal subchondral signal abnormality within the femoral heads. Infection, traumatic contusions, and stress reactions could be considered but are extremely unlikely given the bilateral, symmetric nature of the findings.

Teaching Points

▶ Transient bone marrow edema, previously known as transient osteoporosis, is a condition of unknown etiology.
▶ It most commonly affects the hips but has been described in other locations as well, such as the knees and feet.
▶ It is a self-limited disease that begins with the spontaneous onset of unilateral or bilateral hip pain and typically resolves over a course of 3 to 12 months.
▶ Radiographs may demonstrate regional osteopenia but are often normal.
▶ MR imaging is usually diagnostic and demonstrates diffuse, edema-like signal throughout the marrow of the femoral head and neck without evidence of a fracture line or focus of necrosis. MR findings tend to fade along with the patient's symptoms.

Management

Supportive measures (pain medication, limited weightbearing) may help in the early stages of the disease, and some have reported benefits of bisphosphonate administration. Biopsy or other invasive procedures should be avoided.

Further Readings

Korompilias AV, Karantanas AH, Lykissas MG, Beris AE. Bone marrow edema syndrome. *Skeletal Radiol* 2009;38;425–436.

History

▶ 49-year-old woman with elevated serum calcium level.

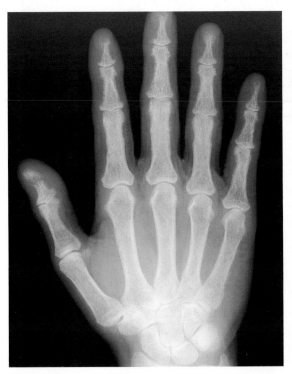

Figure 125.1

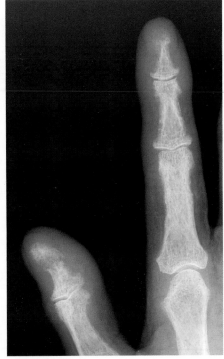

Figure 125.2

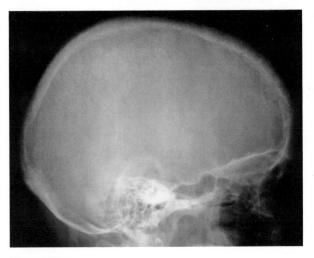

Figure 125.3

Case 125   Primary hyperparathyroidism

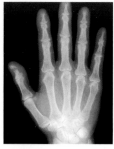

Figure 125.4

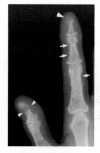

Figure 125.5

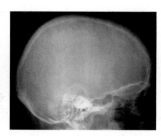

Figure 125.6

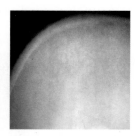

Figure 125.7

Findings

PA image of the hand (Fig. 125.4) and coned-down view of the thumb and index finger (Fig. 125.5) demonstrate areas of prominent subperiosteal resorption in the index finger (*arrows*) and acro-osteolysis of its distal tuft (*large arrowhead*). Additional band-like osteolysis is present in the distal phalanx of the thumb (*small arrowheads*). Lateral (Fig. 125.6) and coned-down lateral (Fig. 125.7) views of the skull show numerous punctuate lucencies in the parietal and parieto-occipital regions, producing a "salt-and-pepper" appearance of the calvarium.

Differential Diagnosis

Secondary hyperparathyroidism (typically related to renal failure—"renal osteodystrophy")

Teaching Points

▸ Primary hyperparathyroidism is typically the result of one or more hyperfunctioning parathyroid adenomas.
▸ The production of excess parathormone triggers extensive osteoclastic activity, resulting in recognizable changes on radiographs.
▸ The most common radiographic findings include diffuse osteopenia and areas of bone resorption, typically in a subperiosteal location, as in this case.
▸ Frequent sites of involvement include the radial aspects of the middle phalanges of the index and long fingers, distal phalangeal tufts (acro-osteolysis), distal end of the clavicle, and symphysis pubis.
▸ Brown tumors are rare. They are statistically more common with primary hyperparathyroidism, but because the secondary form is so much more common clinically, (typically in patients with chronic renal failure), these lesions are more often seen with that form.

Management

Conservative measures, including treatment with bone-forming agents, may be pursued in asymptomatic patients. Surgical removal of the overfunctioning glands is often required.

Further Readings

Fraser WD. Hyperparathyroidism. *Lancet* 2009;*11*:145–153.

History

▶ History of hip discomfort and decreased range of motion in a patient with a 12-year history of hemodialysis for chronic renal failure.

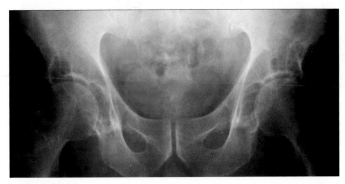

Figure 126.1

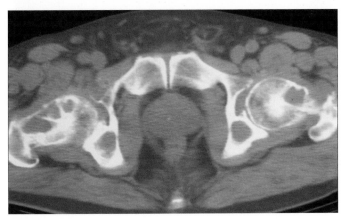

Figure 126.2

Case 126 Amyloidosis (dialysis-related)

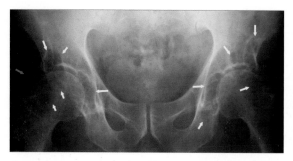

Figure 126.3

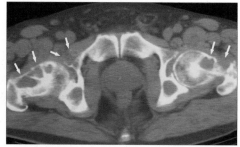

Figure 126.4

Findings

Figures 126.3 and 126.4 (AP radiograph and axial CT of the hips) show multiple well-defined subchondral lucencies with sclerotic rims, better seen on CT, involving the acetabula and subcapital femoral regions of both hips (*white arrows*). Some soft tissue prominence is suggested over the right femoral neck (*gray arrow*). Joint spaces are preserved.

Differential Diagnosis

"Cystic" rheumatoid arthritis; pigmented villonodular synovitis; infection; osteoarthritis

Teaching Points

- ▶ Amyloid arthropathy is characterized by the deposition of beta-2 microglobulin amyloid (Congo red on histology) within bone and soft tissues. It can be primary or secondary, heredofamilial, senile, or localized. The secondary type is most commonly associated with chronic renal disease—that is, a patient who has been on hemodialysis for 10 years or longer ("dialysis-related amyloid arthropathy"), as in this case.
- ▶ Common sites of involvement are hips, wrists, shoulders, knees, and spine.
- ▶ Imaging characteristics of amyloid deposition include the following:
  - ▪ Periarticular well-defined subchondral lucencies occurring on both sides of joints
  - ▪ Multiple sites and typically bilateral (unlike unilateral gout or infection)
  - ▪ No joint-space narrowing (unlike rheumatoid arthritis or osteoarthritis)
  - ▪ No bone production
  - ▪ Soft tissue masses or bursitis often present
  - ▪ Can lead to a destructive spondyloarthropahty as well as carpal tunnel syndrome due to deposition in that region
  - ▪ MR imaging provides the best overall evaluation of the osseous, periarticular and soft tissue changes. Lesions typically demonstrate low signal intensity on T1-weighted images and low to intermediate signal on T2-weighted images, a feature that helps to limit the differential diagnosis in these cases.
  - ▪ Patient can have hepato- or spenomegaly or cardiac abnormalities.

Management

MR is useful in complex cases to differentiate it from other entities in the differential diagnosis, but biopsy is still required for a specific diagnosis.

Further Readings

Kiss E, Keusch G, Zanetti M, Jung T, Schwarz A, Schocke M, Werner J, et al. Dialysis-related amyloidosis revisited. *AJR Am J Roentgenol* 2005;185(6):1460–1467.

History

▶ 17-year-old boy with history of renal failure

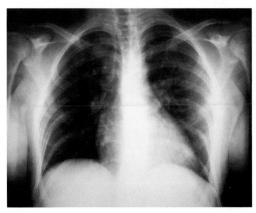

Figure 127.1

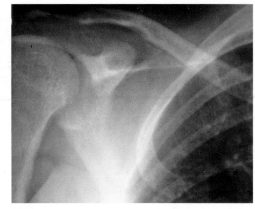

Figure 127.2

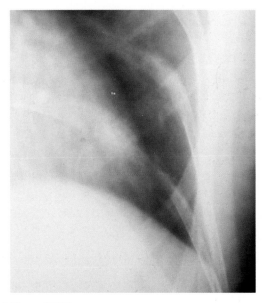

Figure 127.3

Case 127 Renal osteodystrophy

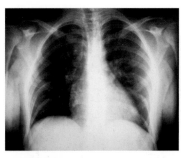

Figure 127.4

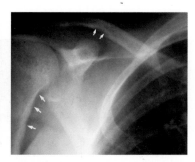

Figure 127.5

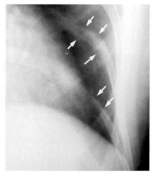

Figure 127.6

Findings

Figure 127.4 (PA view of the chest) reveals an enlarged cardiac silhouette and osseous abnormalities, better shown on coned-down view (Fig. 127.5). Coned-down view of the right shoulder better demonstrates prominent subperiosteal resorption of the proximal humerus (*large arrows*) and subligamentous resorption along the undersurface of the clavicle at the site of attachment of the coracoclavicular ligaments (*small arrows*). Figure 127.6 (coned-down view of the left ribs) reveals additional subperiosteal resorption along the rib margins (*arrows*).

Differential Diagnosis

Primary hyperparathyroidism

Teaching Points

▶ Renal osteodystrophy refers to a group of conditions resulting from abnormal calcium and phosphate metabolism that arise from chronic renal failure.

▶ Associated secondary hyperparathyroidism results in increased parathormone production, which produces osteoclastic resorption of bone, typically in the form of subperiosteal resorption. This often occurs in the phalanges of the hands, along the concave margins of long bones, and at the attachment sites (entheses) of tendons and ligaments.

▶ Osteomalacia may also be associated with renal insufficiency and results in abnormal mineralization, which is manifest as osteopenia, poor corticomedullary differentiation, coarsened, "fuzzy" trabeculae, and occasionally lucent pseudofractures (Looser's zones).

▶ Increased vascular and soft tissue calcifications are commonly seen in these patients as well.

Management

Maintenance of serum calcium and phosphate levels. Calcium and vitamin D supplementation. Dialysis and, if possible, renal transplantation.

Further Readings

Jevtic V. Imaging of renal osteodystrophy. *Eur J Radiol* 2003;46:85–95.

Murphey MD, Sartoris DJ, Quale JL, Pathria MN, Martin NL. Musculoskeletal manifestations of chronic renal insufficiency. *Radiographics* 1993;13:357–379.

History

▶ Left femoral and back pain in a 59-year-old woman

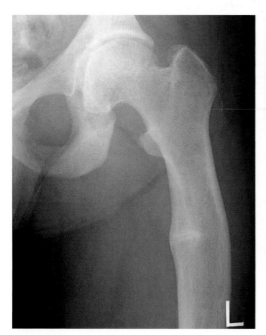

Figure 128.1

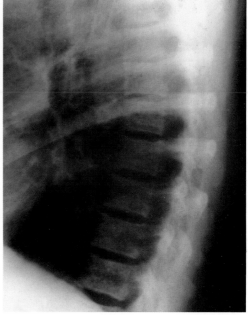

Figure 128.2

Case 128   Osteomalacia

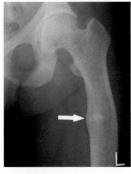

Figure 128.3

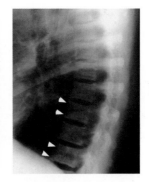

Figure 128.4

Findings

Figure 128.3 (AP radiograph of the left hip) demonstrates diffuse osteopenia. A transverse medial subtrochanteric left femoral cortical lucency with minimal adjacent sclerosis (*white arrows*) is characteristic of a pseudofracture or Looser's zone. Figure 128.4 (lateral radiograph of the spine) demonstrates a coarsened and indistinct trabecular bandlike "rugger jersey" pattern throughout the spine (*arrowheads*) without acute fracture.

Differential Diagnosis

Drug-induced osteomalacia; oncogenic osteomalacia; renal osteodystrophy or hyperparathyroidism; osteoporosis; not Paget disease because of the medial location of the femoral abnormality.

Teaching Points

► Osteomalacia results from inadequate or delayed mineralization of osteoid in mature bone. If this occurs in growing bones, rickets results.

► There are three causes of osteomalacia:

   1. Abnormality of vitamin D metabolism (intake, intestinal, renal or liver)

   2. Abnormality of calcium and phosphorus metabolism

   3. Disorders with no primary abnormalities in vitamin D or mineral metabolism

► Osteopenia is a general and nonspecific finding. Coarsened and indistinct trabeculae occur from bone resorption and deposition and help to distinguish osteomalacia from osteoporosis.

► Looser's zones (pseudofractures caused by deposition of uncalcified osteoid) are characteristic and occur within the medial subtrochanteric femur, pubic rami, axillary margins of the scapula and ribs and posterior proximal ulnae. The medial location in long bones helps differentiate it from the "banana type" fracture of Paget disease found on the convex lateral aspect of long bone andfractures of fibrous dysplasia.

► Coarse indistinct bone is apparent, particularly in the spine, giving a "rugger jersey" appearance, particularly in renal osteodystrophy.

Management

The underlying cause of osteomalacia must be determined. Hand and spine radiographs are useful to help determine the underlying disease process, along with biochemistry and laboratory tests. Medications such as anticonvulsants and bisphosponates for osteoporosis or Paget's disease, as well as tumors, can cause osteomalacia and should be considered.

Further Readings

Pitt M. Rickets and osteomalacia. In *Diagnosis of Bone and Joint Disorders*, 3rd ed. Philadelphia: WB Saunders,1995:1885–1922.

Weissman B, ed. *Imaging of Arthritis and Metabolic Bone Disease*,1st ed. Philadelphia: Saunders Elsevier, 2009:642–678.

History

▶ 32-year-old woman with knee pain status post trauma

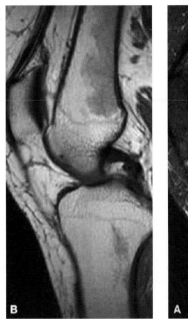

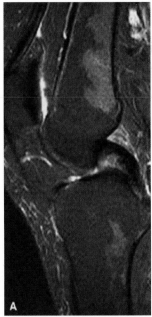

Figure 129.1

Figure 129.2

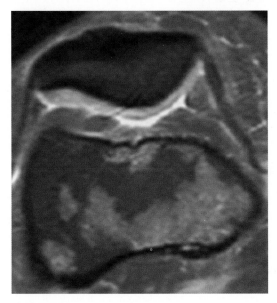

Figure 129.3

Case 129 Hematopoietic marrow (red marrow reconversion)

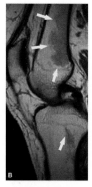
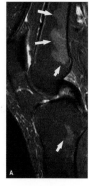
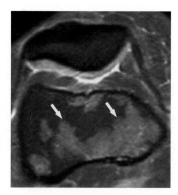

Figure 129.4   **Figure 129.5**   **Figure 129.6**

Findings

Figure 129.4 (T1-weighted sagittal MR) and Figures 129.5 and 129.6 (STIR sagittal and axial T2-weighted fat-saturated MR) show diffuse homogeneous lobular metadiaphyseal marrow signal changes (*white arrows*) within both the femur and tibia that spare the epiphysis. Areas of marrow signal abnormality demonstrate intermediate signal intensity on T1-weighted images and high signal intensity on T2-weighted fat-saturated sequences. No adjacent soft tissue or cortical changes are seen.

Differential Diagnosis

Pathognomonic but must exclude: metastatic disease; myeloma; Gaucher's disease; glycogen storage disease; lymphoma

Teaching Points

▶ Red marrow is hematopoietically active and present throughout the skeleton in childhood but is normally replaced by inactive yellow marrow as the skeleton matures. This process should be complete by the third decade.

▶ With stress, reconversion to red marrow can occur typically within the diametaphysis, with sparing of the epiphysis.

▶ Precursors or stressors for red marrow reconversion include long-term smoking history, anemia, obesity, and long-distance running (marathon runners).

▶ It is more common in women, particularly those of menstruating age.

▶ This benign marrow change can be distinguished from other causes such as infiltrative marrow disease by the following:
  – Follows the anatomic pattern of marrow change in reverse order (diaphysis to articular ends; spares epiphysis)
  – Symmetric and bilateral; no destruction; no enlargement
  – Enhances less than pathologically infiltrated marrow
  – Although it appears relatively bright on fat-saturated T2-weighted images, a key feature is that its signal intensity is brighter than that of muscle on T1-weighted images (unlike most tumors)

Management

If the classic MR findings are present, clinical follow-up is usually sufficient.

Further Readings

Poulton TB, Murphy WD, Wuerk J, Chapek CC, Feiglin DH. Bone marrow reconversion in adults who are smokers: MR imaging findings. *AJR Am J Roentgenol* 1993;*161*(6):1217–1221.

Shellock FG, Morris E, Deutsch AL, et al. Hematopoietic bone marrow hyperplasia: high prevalence on MR images of the knee in asymptomatic marathon runners. *AJR Am J Roentgenol* 1992;*158*:335–338.

Wilson AJ, Hodge J, Pilgram TK, Kang EH, Murphy WA. Prevalence of red marrow around the knee joint in adults as demonstrated on magnetic resonance imaging. *Acad Radiol* 1996;3(7):550–555.

History

▶ Knee pain

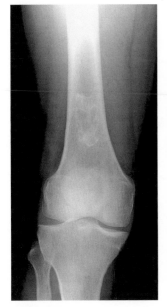

Figure 130.1

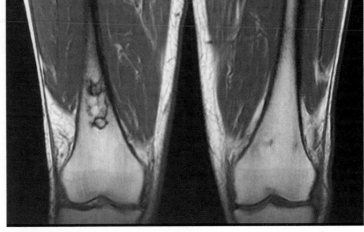

Figure 130.2

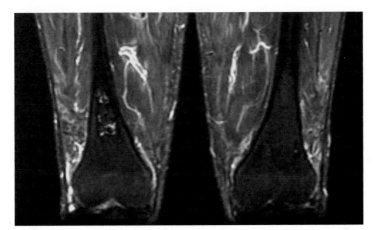

Figure 130.3

Case 130   Medullary infarct

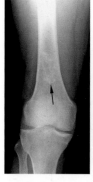
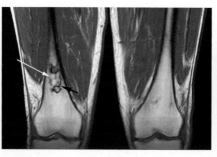
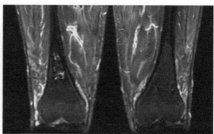

Figure 130.4   **Figure 130.5**   **Figure 130.6**

Findings

Figure 130.4 (AP radiograph) shows a lesion with coarse, curvilinear calcifications in the distal femoral shaft with a thin, sclerotic margin (*arrow*). Figure 130.5 (T1-weighted coronal image) displays a heterogeneous lesion in the marrow of distal femoral shaft. Note the abundant areas of high signal intensity fat within it (*thin arrow*), which are confirmed to be fat by their suppression on the coronal STIR image (Fig. 130.6), as well as the serpentine, low-signal-intensity margin corresponding to the sclerotic border present on the radiographs (*short arrow*). Figure 130.6 (STIR coronal image) demonstrates suppressed fat as well as other nonfatty elements within the area of infarction.

Differential Diagnosis

Radiography: chondroid lesion; MR imaging: none (pathognomonic appearance)

Teaching Points

▶ When visible on radiographs, medullary bone infarctions typically demonstrate coarse calcifications that may be indistinguishable from the "arc and ring" calcifications present in a chondroid tumor.

▶ A thin sclerotic border, as demonstrated in this case, is very suggestive of a medullary infarct (although it is not always present).

▶ MR imaging allows for a confident diagnosis. Diagnostic features include a well-circumscribed lesion with a serpentine, low-signal-intensity border, and areas of fat signal intensity within it.

Management

No specific treatment is required.

Further Readings

Hara H, Akisue T, Fujimoto T, et. al. Magnetic resonance imaging of medullary bone infarction in the early stage. Clinical Imaging 2008;32:147–151.

History

▶ Acute onset of back pain without history of trauma

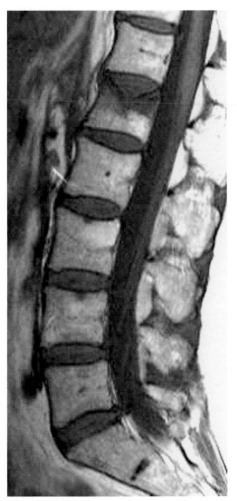

Figure 131.1

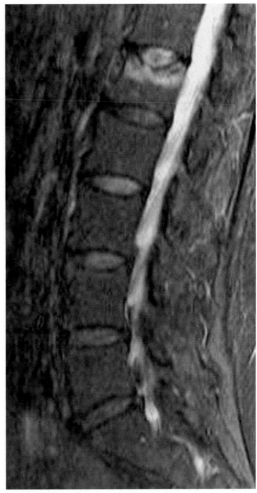

Figure 131.2

Case 131 Osteoporotic vertebral insufficiency fracture

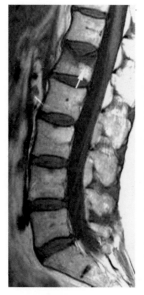

Figure 131.3

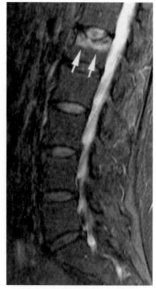

Figure 131.4

Findings

Sagittal T1-weighted (Fig. 131.3) and STIR (Fig. 131.4) images demonstrate a superior endplate compression fracture of the L1 vertebral body with associated edema-like signal abnormality within the adjacent marrow. Note the sharp demarcation between the normal and abnormal marrow signal (*arrows*).

Differential Diagnosis

Pathologic fracture secondary to underlying tumor

Teaching Points

▸ An atraumatic vertebral fracture is usually due to underlying malignancy or osteoporosis.
▸ Radiography and radionuclide bone scanning demonstrate nonspecific osteopenia and increased activity, respectively, but are otherwise unrevealing as to the exact etiology. Because MR imaging can directly display the underlying marrow, it is often able to provide a more specific diagnosis.
▸ MR findings suggestive of a malignant etiology include abnormal signal replacing the entire vertebral body, absence of a fracture line, bowing of the posterior vertebral cortex, and abnormal epidural or paraspinous tissue.
▸ Findings suggesting a benign etiology include partial replacement of the vertebral marrow with a sharp border between the normal and abnormal signal intensity (as illustrated in this case), a discrete fracture line, and a lack of abnormal epidural or paraspinous soft tissue.
▸ In those cases that demonstrate ambiguous or indeterminate findings, either a short-term follow-up MRI (to look for evidence of healing in the case of an osteoporotic fracture) or biopsy should be obtained.

Management

Usually conservative (rest, analgesics); vertebroplasty/kyphoplasty; rarely surgery

Further Readings

Jung H-S, Jee W-H, McCauley TR, Ha K-Y, Choi K-H. Discrimination of metastatic from acute osteoporotic compression spinal fractures with MR imaging. *Radiographics* 2003;23:179–187.

History

▶ 45-year-old woman weighing 94 lbs with hip pain and malaise

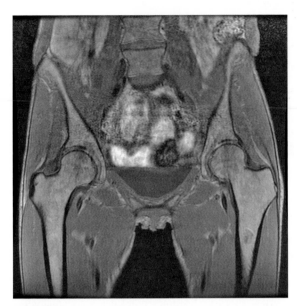

Figure 132.1

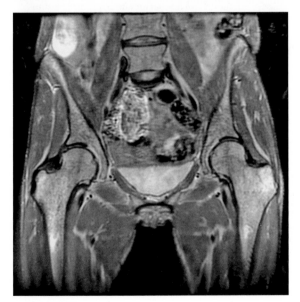

Figure 132.2

Case 132   Anorexia nervosa (chronic malnutrition and marrow changes)

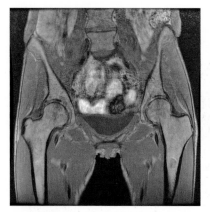

Figure 132.3

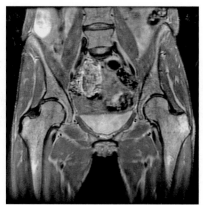

Figure 132.4

Findings

Figures 132.3 and 132.4 (Coronal T1and STIR MR images) show diffuse abnormal intermediate-low (T1)/and intermediate-high (STIR) marrow signal with STIR marrow slightly brighter than on the T1 images. There is near-complete loss of subcutaneous fat. DXA (not shown) demonstrated marked osteoporosis.

Differential Diagnosis

Causes of serous atrophy; aplastic anemia; infiltrative marrow disorders (Erlenmeyer flask deformity); multiple stress fractures; marrow reconversion (proximal to distal); diffuse sarcoidosis

Teaching Points

▶ Marrow changes in anorexia nervosa are attributable to early osteoporosis and premature conversion of red marrow to yellow marrow in a distal-to-proximal manner.

▶ "Serous atrophy" (increased free water = increased signal intensity on MR) refers to gelatinous transformation of bone marrow (fat cell atrophy, loss of hematopoietic cells, and deposition of extracellular substances). It is a sign of a generalized severe illness also seen in alcoholism, malignancy, or chronic heart disease.

▶ MR marrow: low signal intensity on T1, high on T2/STIR. This may mask stress fractures. Rarely, there is diffuse increased T1 signal intensity marrow.

▶ A clue is reduced or no fat signal marrow on T1 with loss of subcutaneous fat more so than abdominal fat in a patient with severely low weight.

Management

Imaging is the mainstay for diagnosis and treatment. MR and Tc99 bone scan are useful in patients with severe progression of disease or increased pain or muscle symptoms, with the latter helpful in fracture detection. Treatment involves glucocorticosteroids and methotrexate. DXA should be performed to determine bone mineral density (BMD), as a low BMD and vitamin D/calcium balance disruption has been reported as a potential complication.

Further Readings

Ecklund K, Valapeyam S, Feldman HA, et al. Bone marrow changes in adolescent girls with anorexia nervosa. *J Bone Miner Res* 2010;*25*:298–304.

Vande Berg BC, Malghem J, Devuyst O, Maldaque BE, Lambert MJ. Anorexia nervosa: correlation between MR appearance of bone marrow and severity of disease. *Radiology* 1994;*193*:859–864.

Vande Berg BC, Malghem J, Lecouvet FE, Lambert M, Maldague BE. Distribution of serouslike bone marrow changes in the lower limbs of patients with anorexia nervosa. *AJR Am J Roentgenol* 1996;*166*:621–625.

History

▶ Acute knee pain

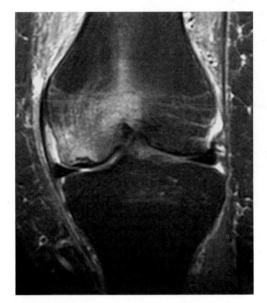

Figure 133.1

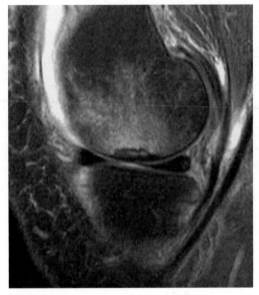

Figure 133.2

Case 133 Subchondral femoral insufficiency fracture ("spontaneous osteonecrosis")

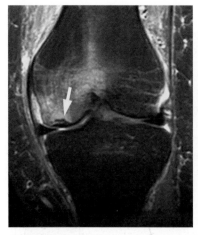

Figure 133.3

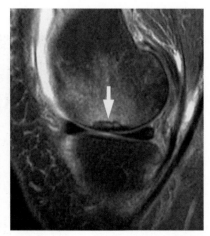

Figure 133.4

Findings

Figure 133.3 (coronal STIR image) shows extensive, abnormal edema-like signal intensity within the medial femoral condyle as well as a small low-signal-intensity subchondral fracture line (*arrow*). Figure 133.4 (sagittal STIR image) again demonstrates the morphology of the insufficiency fracture that parallels the subchondral plate of the condyle (*arrow*).

Differential Diagnosis

None

Teaching Points

- ► "Spontaneous osteonecrosis" of the knee is a misnomer in that it is a painful condition of the knee that results from a subchondral insufficiency fracture, typically involving the weightbearing portion of the medial femoral condyle, although other sites, such as the lateral femoral condyle or proximal tibia, may be affected.
- ► It typically occurs in older patients who describe an acute onset of knee pain.
- ► Radiographs are usually normal in the early stages but may reveal a focus of subchondral collapse if the lesion progresses.
- ► The most conspicuous finding on MR imaging is widespread edema-like signal throughout the marrow of the medial femoral condyle, usually much more extensive than what is seen with a posttraumatic contusion.
- ► Careful inspection of the subchondral region will reveal a curvilinear low-signal fracture line that parallels the articular surface of the bone.

Management

This entity may be managed conservatively (protected weightbearing, etc.) or with surgery such as a core decompression, osteochondral autograft transfer, tibial osteotomy or knee arthroplasty (unicondylar arthroplasty in earlier stages or total joint replacement if there has been significant joint degeneration).

Further Readings

Kattapuram TM, Kattapuram SV. Spontaneous osteonecrosis of the knee. *Eur J Radiol* 2008;67:42–48.

Yamamoto T, Bullough PG. Spontaneous osteonecrosis of the knee: the result of subchondral insufficiency fracture. *J Bone Joint Surg Am* 2000;82:858–866.

History

▶ Knee pain. No history of acute injury.

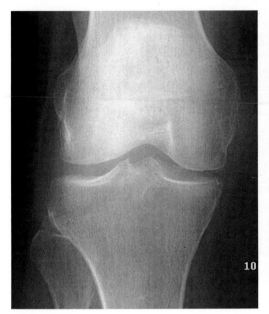

Figure 134.1

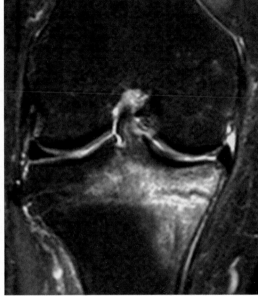

Figure 134.2

Case 134 Insufficiency fracture of the tibia

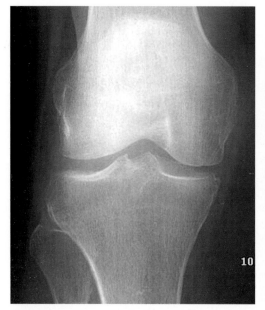

Figure 134.3

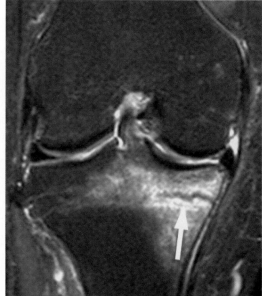

Figure 134.4

Findings

Figure 134.3 (initial PA radiograph of the knee) demonstrates diffuse osteopenia but is otherwise normal. Figure 134.4 (coronal STIR image) reveals an incomplete, transverse fracture of the medial tibial plateau (*arrow*).

Differential Diagnosis

None

Teaching Points

▸ Chronic repetitive stresses applied to bone result in a spectrum of injuries ranging from microfractures and increased bone turnover ("stress reaction") to a mechanical failure of the bone ("stress fracture").

▸ Radiographs are very insensitive in detecting these injuries, especially in their early stages. There are some reports that the sensitivity of radiography may be as low as 15% at the time of clinical presentation.

▸ Bone scan will demonstrate foci of increased uptake at these sites, but MRI is thought to be just as sensitive and provides the added advantage of improved specificity. This is especially true in older patients, who may present with atraumatic musculoskeletal pain, in which the primary differential considerations are tumor versus insufficiency fracture.

▸ By demonstrating the associated marrow edema and hemorrhage (high signal on fluid-sensitive sequences) and an associated fracture line, as in this case, a specific diagnosis can be made.

▸ Prompt, accurate diagnosis is essential to avoid the morbidity of developing a displaced fracture.

Management

Conservative measures such as protected weightbearing and pain medication are typically all that are required.

Further Readings

Krestan C, Hoijreh A. Imaging of insufficiency fractures. *Eur J Radiol* 2009;71:398–405.

History

▶ 70-year-old man with history of left hip deformity and mild pain

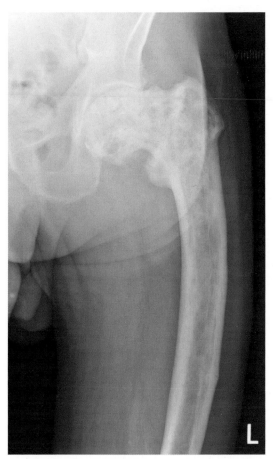

Figure 135.1

Case 135 Paget-related insufficiency fracture of the femoral diaphysis

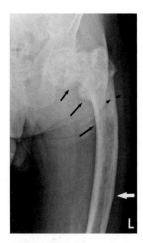

Figure 135.2

Findings

Figure 135.2 (AP radiograph of the proximal left femur) demonstrates coxa vara deformity of the proximal femur (*black arrows*) with lateral diametaphyseal bowing, cortical thickening (*arrowheads*), trabecular prominence, and a subtle incomplete linear lucency (*white arrow*) through the lateral proximal femoral cortex and lateral intramedullary femoral diaphysis.

Differential Diagnosis

Pathognomonic for Paget-related insufficiency fracture

Teaching Points

▸ Paget disease occurs in 3% to 4% of the population over 40 years of age and is characterized by lytic, mixed, and osteoblastic phases and progressive osteoclastic and osteoblastic activity. This activity leads to not only enlargement of bone but also weakening of bone.

▸ Fractures (insufficiency type) are the most common complication of Paget's disease. Common locations for Paget-related insufficiency fractures include the femur, tibia, humerus, pelvis, and spine.

▸ Subtrochanteric femoral fractures are most common and occur in patients with longstanding disease (F > M).

▸ Fractures occur initially as incomplete fractures on the convex surfaces of the long bones (unlike osteomalacia Looser's zones, which occur on the concave surface of bone) and eventually become complete in nature, referred to as "banana" fractures.

▸ Other complications of Paget disease include arthritis, neurologic symptoms, and neoplastic transformation (1%).

Management

Close radiographic follow-up of Paget-related insufficiency fractures is recommended to preclude progression to complete fracture. Orthopedic intervention may be required for stabilization. If the area of lucency becomes irregular or pain increases, advanced imaging (CT or MRI) may be of benefit to exclude secondary malignancy or possible pathologic fracture in these patients.

Further Readings

Smith SE, Murphy MD, Motamedi K, Mulligan ME, Resnik CS, Gannon F. From the Archives of the AFIP: Radiologic spectrum of Paget disease of bone and its complications with pathologic correlation. *Radiographics* 2002;*22*:1191–1216.
Theodorou DJ, Theodorou SJ, Kakitsubata Y. Imaging of Paget disease of bone and its musculoskeletal complications: Review. *AJR Integrated Imaging* 2011;*196*(6):S64–S75.

History

► Bilateral hip pain

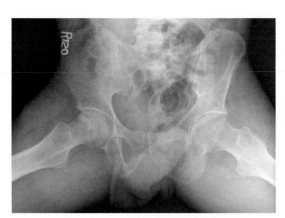

Figure 136.1

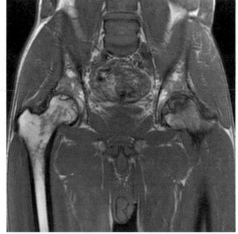

Figure 136.2

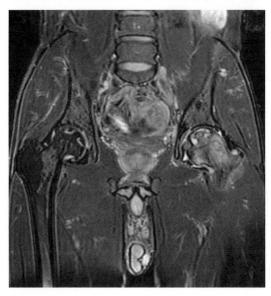

Figure 136.3

Case 136 Avascular necrosis, bilateral hips

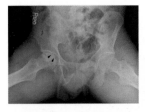 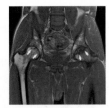 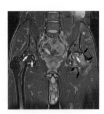

Figure 136.4   **Figure 136.5**   **Figure 136.6**

Findings

Radiograph (Fig. 136.4) shows mild increased sclerosis of the right femoral head with subtle crescentic luceny and mild cortical discontinuity in the subcortical region (*black arrowheads*). T1-weighted coronal MR image (second patient; Fig. 136.5) shows subchondral areas of abnormal serpentine low signal intensity within both femoral heads (*white arrows*) with low-signal-intensity marrow change in the left femoral head/neck. No fracture, effusion, or cortical collapse is seen. T2-weighted fat-saturated coronal MR image (Fig. 136.6) shows serpentine "double-line" signs—low signal intensity in close proximity to a line of high signal intensity—right great than left, in the femoral heads (*white arrows*). There is mild marrow edema of the left femoral head/neck with a small effusion (*black arrows*).

Differential Diagnosis

Classic appearance on MR. No differential diagnosis.

Teaching Points

▶ Avascular necrosis (aseptic necrosis or ischemic necrosis) refers to ischemic death within bone and marrow of the epiphysis or subarticular region. If this occurs in the metadiaphyseal region, it is called a medullary infarction.
▶ Location: femoral head > humeral heads > distal femur > proximal tibia. Increased risk of contralateral involvement
▶ Causes: long-term steroid use, trauma with disruption of vascular supply (femoral neck fracture), hemoglobinopathies, sickle cell anemia, alcoholism, post transplant, radiation, pancreatitis, idiopathic
▶ Radiographic staging is important for treatment.
  ▪ *Stage 3: Crescent sign* (subchondral lucency) and subchondral collapse signifies advanced disease without flattened femoral head on radiographs. These changes are best demonstrated on a frog-lateral view.
  ▪ *Stage 4:* Flattened femoral head with cortical collapse and normal joint space
▶ Tc99m: Uptake in area of necrosis before radiographic abnormalities
▶ CT and radiography: Early femoral head sclerosis, eventual crescent sign, collapse of femoral head
▶ MR: More sensitive than radiographs, CT, or scintigraphy. Low signal-intensity serpentine lines are typically seen on T1 and the classic *double-line* sign (see above) is present on T2-weighted images in 80% of cases. Edema within femoral.

Management

Treatment is dependent on stage of disease. Conservative therapy includes limited weight bearing, immobilization and pain medication. Bisphosphonates and statins have shown promise in delaying disease progression. Advanced disease may require surgical intervention: Core decompression with or without bone grafts, osteotomy, electrical treatments, and eventual joint replacement

Further Readings

Beltran J et al. Femoral head avascular necrosis: MR imaging with clinical pathologic and radionuclide correlation. *Radiology* 1988;*166*:215–220.
Mitchell GD et al. Femoral head avascular necrosis: correlation with MR imaging radiographic staging, radionuclide imaging and clinical findings. *Radiology 162*;1987:709–715.

History

▶ 22-year-old man with history of previous radiation therapy T12-S2 for spinal ependymoma

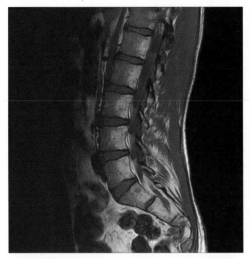

Figure 137.1

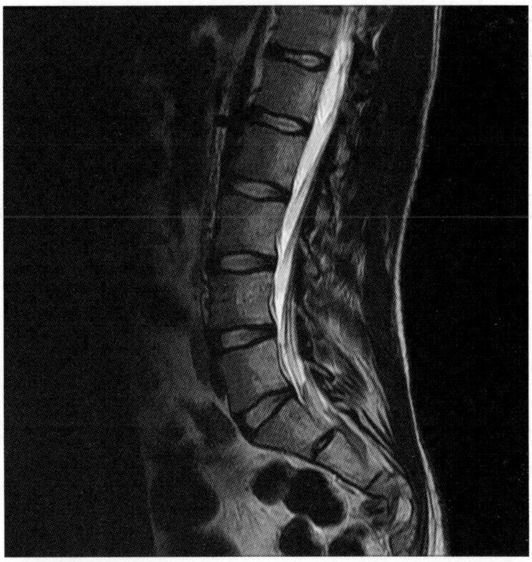

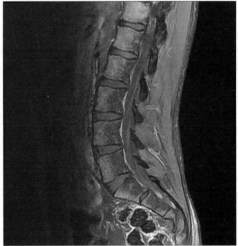

Figure 137.2

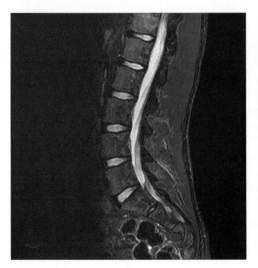

Figure 137.3

Figure 137.4

Case 137 Postradiation marrow changes

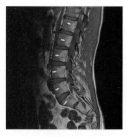
Figure 137.5

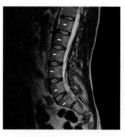
Figure 137.6

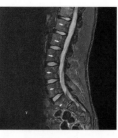
Figure 137.7

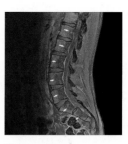
Figure 137.8

Findings

Figure 137.5 (T1-weighted sagittal image) and Figures 137.6 and 137.7 (Sagittal T2-weighted and STIR images) show well-demarcated vertical fatty marrow change throughout the entire posterior lumbar spine and upper sacrum (*white arrows*) (high [T1,T2]/low [STIR]). Figure 137.8 (T1-weighted FS post-gadolinium image) demonstrates decreased enhancement in the posterior half of the vertebral bodies (*white arrows*), reflecting the borders of the radiation portal.

Differential Diagnosis

Pathognomonic for postradiation portal marrow changes. Differential diagnosis: fatty age-related marrow changes or hemangioma, but the well-demarcated margins and multilevel involvement make these unlikely.

Teaching Points

▶ MR is the best modality for assessing postradiation marrow changes.
▶ The marrow in the radiation portal undergoes fatty transformation conforming to the portal, resulting in high-intensity T1 marrow signal similar to that of subcutaneous fat.
▶ Typically homogeneous—if heterogeneous or focal lesions, think residual or current marrow disease, marrow recoversion with GCRC therapy (if nodular), secondary malignancy, metastasis, or fracture.
▶ MR marrow appearance is dependent on timing—acute versus chronic
  ▪ STIR signal: high acute, low chronic
  ▪ Enhancement: prominent acute (vascular congestion), none chronic
▶ Dose-dependent fatty radiation marrow changes
  ▪ 50 Gy—persist for years
  ▪ 20 to 30 Gy—may return to normal after 10 years
▶ Tc99m sulfur colloid scan—sharply demarcated focal or diffuse photopenic region represents radiation therapy portal.
▶ PET FDG18—decreased marrow metabolic activity shown in the area of marrow change.

Management

Complications of postradiation therapy include insufficiency fractures, compression fractures of the spine, postradiation myelitis, necrosis, and secondary osteosarcoma. Careful MR assessment before contrast (T2 FS, STIR, T1) and after contrast (T1 FS post) and CT are required to exclude these entities in a patient with new onset of back pain.

Further Readings

Blomlie V et al. Female pelvic bone marrow: serial MR imaging before, during and after radiation therapy. *Radiology* 1995;*194*(2):537–543.
Onu M et al. Early MR changes in vertebral bone marrow for patient following radiotherapy. *Eur Radiol* 2001;*11*(8):1463–1469.
Otake S et al. Radiation-induced changes in MR signal intensity and contrast enhancement of lumbosacral vertebrae: do changes occur only inside the radiation therapy field? *Radiology* 2002;*222*(1):179–183.

Part VII   Pediatric

History

▶ 14-year-old boy with right shoulder pain following trauma

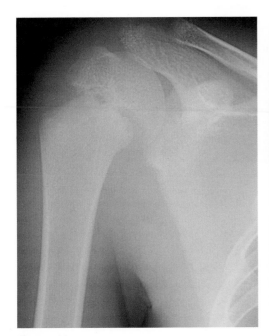

Figure 138.1

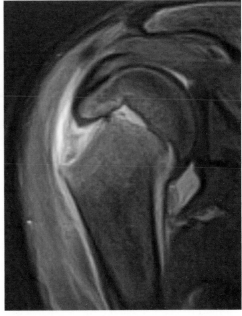

Figure 138.2

Case 138 Salter-Harris type I fracture of the humerus

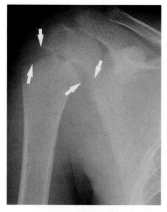

Figure 138.3

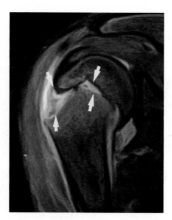

Figure 138.4

Findings

Figure 138.3 (AP radiograph of the right proximal humerus) demonstrates abnormal widening and offset of the proximal humeral growth plate (*white arrows*). Figure 138.4 (coronal STIR image of the proximal right humerus) better demonstrates the disruption of the growth plate (*white arrows*) with posttraumatic fluid within the growth plate, offset of the epiphysis, and surrounding soft tissue edema.

Differential Diagnosis

Usually pathognomonic but could consider infection if no trauma

Teaching Points

- ▶ Salter-Harris fractures refer to injuries involving the epiphyseal plate or growth plate of long bones in skeletally immature patients.
- ▶ Salter-Harris classification Mnemonic (SALTR)
    I.   Transverse fracture through growth plate or physis (epiphyseal slip) (**S**AME)
    II. Epiphyseal plate fracture with extension into the adjacent metaphysis (**A**BOVE)
    III. Fracture through epiphysis extending through epiphyseal plate (most common type; 85%) (**L**OWER)
    IV. Fracture of epiphysis and metaphysis crossing the epiphyseal plate (**T**HROUGH)
    V.   Compression fracture of the epiphyseal plate (**R**AMMED) (**WR**ECKED or **CR**USHED)
- ▶ Majority heal without complication; however, growth plate injuries can lead to growth arrest/shortening due to injury and inhibition of epiphyseal circulation with development of bony bridging at the plate, resulting in abnormal angulation.
- ▶ Growth plates are prone to stress injuries (chronic type I), resulting in widening and irregularity of the growth plate (gymnasts, baseball pitchers, runners).

Management

If a growth plate injury is suspected on radiographs, imaging the opposite joint to confirm asymmetry may be of benefit, and MR or CT is best to evaluate the true extent of the injury.

Further Readings

Manaster BJ, May DA, Disler D. *Musculoskeletal Imaging, The Requisites*, 2nd ed. Philadelphia, PA. Mosby Elsevier Publishing, 2002;188–399.
Rogers LF, Poznanski AK. Imaging of epiphyseal injuries. *Radiology* 1994;*191*:297–308.

Case 139

History

- 4-year-old boy with left shin pain and swelling following injury and 9-year-old girl with left forearm pain and swelling following injury

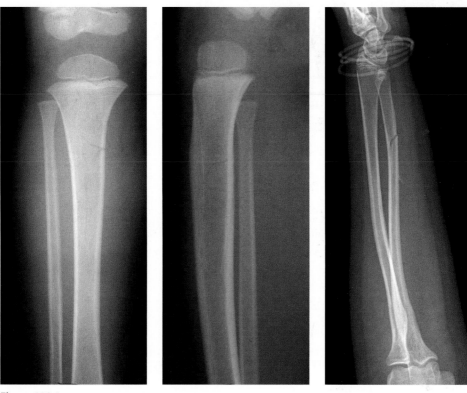

Figure 139.1

Figure 139.2

Figure 139.3

Case 139   Greenstick fracture

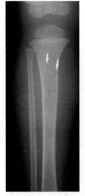 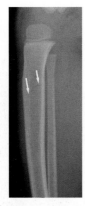 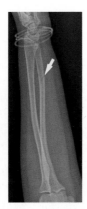

Figure 139.4   **Figure 139.5**   **Figure 139.6**

Findings

Figures 139.4 and 139.5 (AP and lateral radiographs of the left tibia and fibula) show a nondisplaced fracture (*white arrows*) extending from the proximal medial tibial cortex to the mid-tibia without lateral extension. Figure 139.6 (AP view of the left forearm) shows an oblique nondisplaced fracture of the distal medial ulna (*white arrow*) with sparing of the lateral ulnar cortex and radius. Mild ulnar bowing is present.

Differential Diagnosis

Pathognomonic. Must distinguish from the continuum of torus fracture (buckle fracture), transverse fracture, or spiral fracture.

Teaching Points

▶ The greenstick fracture is a nondisplaced or minimally displaced fracture (typically transverse, then extending longitudinally) involving only one cortex, typically of the diaphysis of a long bone with a predilection for the bones of the forearm or lower leg.

▶ Greenstick fractures are considered stable fractures and may have associated bowing of the nonaffected cortex.

▶ They typically occur in the soft growing bones of infants and children secondary to bending forces perpendicular to bone, impaction injury, or a fall from a height.

▶ While nonaccidental trauma may result in a greenstick injury (i.e., blow to the forearm), it more typically causes spiral fractures.

▶ Greenstick fractures may be difficult to visualize on radiographs. CT may be required for confirmation. Sequelae may include post-traumatic cortical defects when the radius is affected.

Management

Removable splint or casting (short- or long-arm types, depending on the presence of displacement). Imaging assessment for involvement of the other bone within the forearm or calf, as this may be present due to impaction forces. Follow-up radiographs to ensure healing and stable position are recommended.

Further Readings

Fayad LM, Corl F, Fishman EK. Pediatric skeletal trauma: use of multiplanar reformatted and three-dimensional 64-row multidetector CT in the emergency department. *Radiographics* 2009;*20*(1):135–150.

Lee P, Hunter TB, Taljanovic M. Musculoskeletal colloquialisms: How did we come up with these names? *Radiographics* 2004;*24*:1009–1027.

Roach R, Cassar-Pullicino V, Summers BN. Pediatric post-traumatic cortical defects of the distal radius. *Pediatr Radiol* 2002;*32*(5):333–339.

History

▶ 12-year-old boy with left hip pain

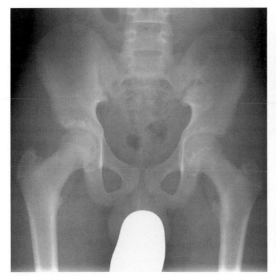

Figure 140.1

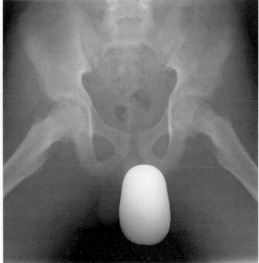

Figure 140.2

Case 140 Slipped capital femoral epiphysis (SCFE), left femur

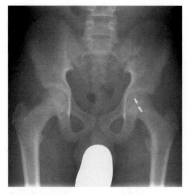

Figure 140.3

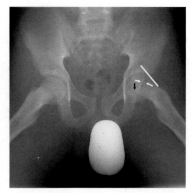

Figure 140.4

Findings

Figure 140.3 (AP view) demonstrates slight widening of the left femoral growth plate (*white arrows*) with mild irregularity of the metaphysis. The epiphysis appears slightly more medial and inferior (*black arrow*) than expected with respect to the lateral femoral neck, which becomes more evident on the frog-leg view (Fig. 140.4). A line (*white line*) drawn along the left lateral femoral neck cortex does NOT intersect with the femoral head as it normally should. There is no evidence of dislocation.

Differential Diagnosis

Healing Salter I fracture; avascular necrosis

Teaching Points

▶ SCFE refers to infero- or postero-medial displacement of the femoral epiphysis with respect to the femoral neck through an open growth plate (between the proliferative and hypertrophic zones).

▶ SCFE is bilateral in 25% to 50% of cases, so it is important to evaluate both hips. Typically presents with a limp or pain in the hip and/or knee.

▶ May be chronic (resulting in more deformity of the head and neck) or acute in nature

▶ Radiographically, SCFE is best seen on frog-leg lateral images with associated irregularity of the femoral metaphysis or widening of the femoral growth plate. Slips may be mild or severe.

▶ Occurs in children (11 years girls, 14 years boys, with a M:F ratio of 2.5:1) just before the closure of the growth plates and is more common in overweight children with mildly delayed skeletal ages

▶ MR may detect early abnormalities of the growth plate prior to radiographic changes (metaphyseal edema on T2 with or without mild displacement).

▶ CT can confirm the inframedial slip of the epiphysis with respect to the femoral neck on axial and coronal images.

Management

MR may be useful in detecting early changes of the growth plate prior to the development of radiographic abnormalities, allowing for earlier treatment. Treatment involves stabilization of the head without anatomic reduction. If not treated, complications include hip dysplasia, early osteoarthritis, and osteonecrosis (more common in acute slips).

Further Readings

Aronsson DD, Loder R, Breur GJ, Weinstein S. Slipped capital femoral epiphysis: current concepts. *J Am Acad Orthop Surg* 2006;*14*(12):666–679.

Umans H, Liebling MS, Moy L, Haramati N, Macy NJ, Pritzker HA. Slipped capital femoral epiphysis: a physeal lesion diagnosed by MRI, with radiographic and CT correlation. *Skeletal Radiol* 1998;*27*:139–144.

History

▶ None

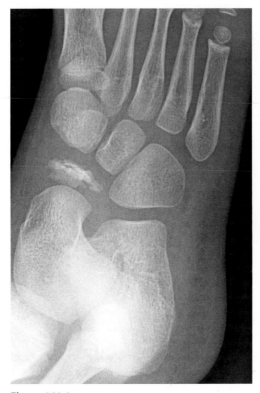

Figure 141.1

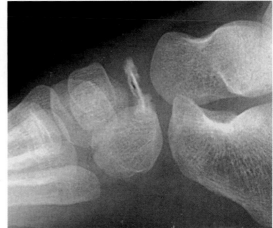

Figure 141.2

Case 141 Osteochondrosis of the tarsal navicular (Kohler's disease)

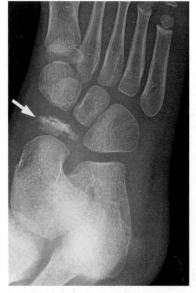

Figure 141.3

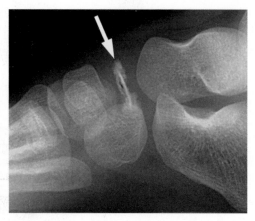

Figure 141.4

Findings

Oblique (Fig. 141.3) and lateral (Fig. 141.4) radiographs of the foot in this skeletally immature patient demonstrate a small, irregular ossification center of the tarsal navicular (*arrows*).

Differential Diagnosis

None

Teaching Points

▶ The osteochondroses are a heterogeneous group of entities that affect the epiphyses and/or apophyses in skeletally immature patients. These include the following:
  - Legg-Calvé-Perthes disease (femoral head)
  - Panner's disease (elbow-capitellum)
  - Osgood-Schlatter disease (tibial tuberosity)
  - Sinding-Larsen-Johansson disease (patella)

▶ Kohler's disease involves the tarsal navicular and often results in a small, irregular ossification center, as in this case.

▶ It may be symptomatic but is self-limited, with the bone returning to a normal appearance within 2 to 4 years. As a result, many believe that this "disease" is likely a normal variation in ossification.

Management

Temporary short walking cast if symptomatic

Further Readings

Borges JL, Guille JT, Bowen JR. Kohler's bone disease of the tarsal navicular. *J Pediatr Orthop* 1995;*15*:596–598.

History

▶ 10-year-old boy with right hip pain

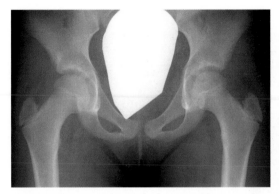

Figure 142.1

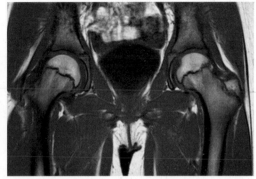

Figure 142.2

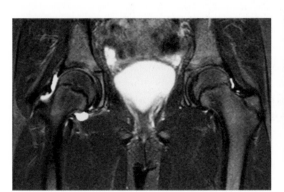

Figure 142.3

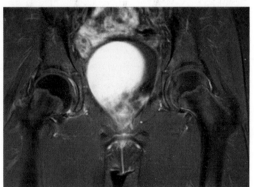

Figure 142.4

Case 142 Ischemia of the right capital femoral epiphysis (early Legg-Perthes disease)

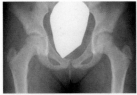

Figure 142.5

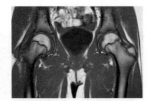

Figure 142.6

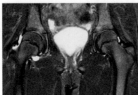

Figure 142.7

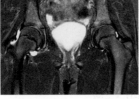

Figure 142.8

Findings

Figure 142.5 (AP radiograph of the pelvis) shows no evidence of right hip pathology. Coronal T1-weighted (Fig. 142.6) and STIR (Fig. 142.7) images of the pelvis reveal a small right hip joint effusion. The capital femoral epiphyses appear normal and symmetric. Figure 142.8 (coronal fat-saturated T1-weighted post-gadolinium image) demonstrates asymmetry of the epiphyses with a diffuse lack of epiphyseal enhancement on the right (*arrow*), compatible with hypoperfusion.

Differential Diagnosis

Pre-contrast images: possible septic right hip joint. Post-contrast image: rarely seen in septic arthritis (see below).

Teaching Points

▸ Idiopathic avascular necrosis of the capital femoral epiphysis (Legg-Calvè-Perthes disease) is a relatively common cause of hip pain in children.

▸ It has a peak incidence at 5 to 6 years of age and affects males more commonly than females (ratio ~5:1).

▸ Radiographs are often normal in the early stages of the disease; epiphyseal fragmentation and collapse are common findings in its later stages.

▸ MR imaging has proven to be exquisitely sensitive for detecting early Legg-Calvè-Perthes disease, especially when combined with intravenous contrast (as in this case), when nonenhanced MR images are normal. However, it must be noted that decreased epiphyseal enhancement has also been described in a small number of patients shown to have a septic hip, so correlation with clinical and laboratory findings is crucial.

▸ In later stages, MR findings include variable, often heterogeneous signal abnormality within the epiphysis on all sequences.

Management

Variable depending on age and stage of disease. Ranges from observation to reconstructive hip surgery.

Further Readings

Dillman JR, Hernandez RJ. MRI of Legg-Calvè-Perthes disease. *AJR Am J Roentgenol* 2009;*193*:1394–1407.
Merlini L, Combescure C, DeRosa V, Anooshiravani, Hanquinet S. Diffusion-weighted imaging findings in Perthes disease with dynamic gadolinium enhance subtracted (DGS) MR correlation: a preliminary study. *Pediatr Radiol* 2010;*40*:318–325.

History

▶ 19-year-old with knee, wrist, and hand pain and swelling for 10 years

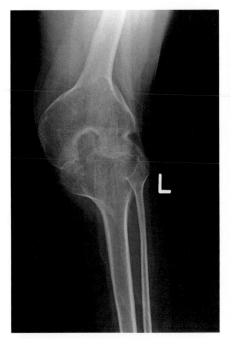

Figure 143.1

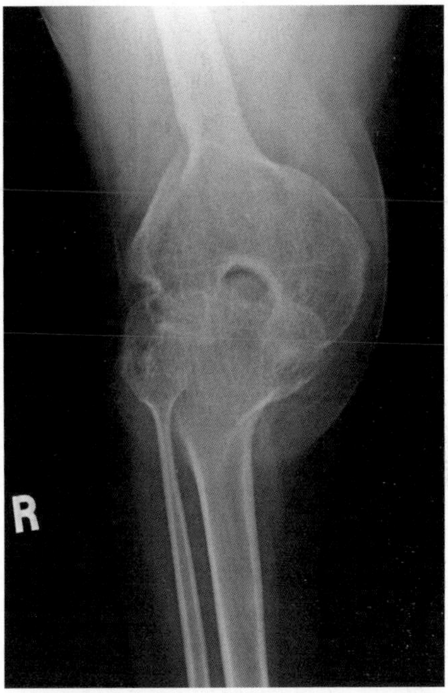

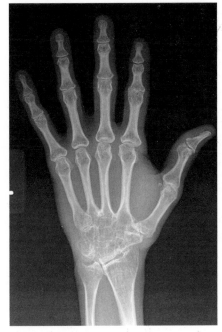

Figure 143.2

Figure 143.3

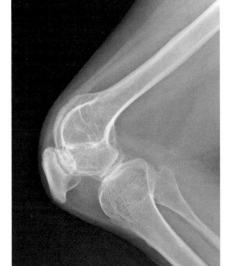

Figure 143.4

Case 143 Juvenile chronic arthritis

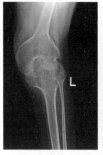
Figure 143.5

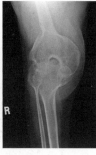
Figure 143.6

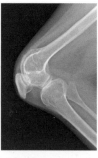
Figure 143.7

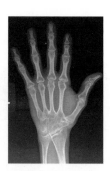
Figure 143.8

Findings

Figures 143.5 through 143.7 (AP bilateral knees and lateral knee) and 143.8 (AP hand and wrist) demonstrate: Gracile bones with epiphyseal overgrowth, symmetric joint space narrowing, and diffuse osteopenia of knees, hands, and wrists, overgrowth and squaring of the patella and widening of the intercondylar notch of the knees and ankylosis of the intercarpal and carpal-metacarpal joints.

Differential Diagnosis

Cerebral palsy or other neuromuscular syndrome; hemophilia

Teaching Points

▶ Juvenile chronic arthritis is defined as a group of systemic inflammatory disorders affecting children under the age of 16; however, some of these cases may not be diagnosed until after 16 years of age, as in this case. Classification includes the following categories:
▶ Juvenile-onset adult type
▶ (Seropositive) rheumatoid arthritis
▶ (Seronegative) chronic arthritis (Still disease)
  ▪ Juvenile-onset ankylosing spondylitis
  ▪ Psoriatic arthritis
  ▪ Arthritis of inflammatory bowel disease
  ▪ Seronegative forms of spondyloarthropathy
▶ Disturbances in enchondral bone formation give rise to metaphyseal and growth plate irregularities.
▶ Overgrowth of the epiphysis occurs secondary to hyperemia.
▶ A widened intercondylar notch of the knee and squaring of the patella are characteristic findings.
▶ Undertubulation of the long bones is secondary to premature growth plate fusion.
▶ Involvement of the wrist and proximal hands predominates, but the disease can involve the hips, knees, and ankles.
▶ Joint space narrowing (symmetric), marginal erosions, soft tissue swelling, and periarticular/diffuse osteoporosis are typical with ankylosis if severe.
▶ Complications include osteoporosis, flexion contractures and deformities, growth retardation (due to early fusion of growth plates), and cervical spine involvement, but 80% of children have resolution of the disease without complications.

Management

NSAIDs, disease-modifying drugs (DMARDs; e.g., methotrexate and immunosuppressive therapies), corticosteroids.

Further Readings

Brower AC, Flemming DJ. *Arthritis in black and white*, 2nd ed. Philadelphia: Saunders, 1997:391–404.
Resnick D. *Diagnosis of bone and joint disorders*, 3rd ed., Vol. 2. Philadelphia: Saunders, 1995:971–991.

History

▸ Intermittent ankle pain and swelling

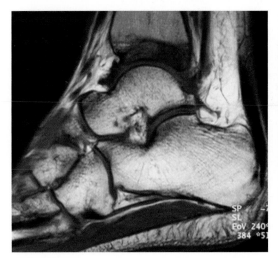

Figure 144.1

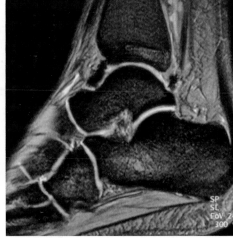

Figure 144.2

Case 144 Hemophilia

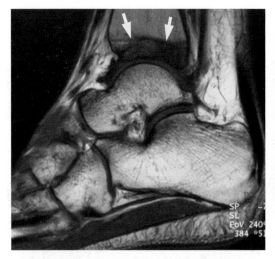

Figure 144.3

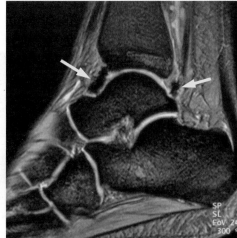

Figure 144.4

Findings

Figure 144.3 (sagittal T1-weighted image) shows extensive low signal throughout the subchondral bone of the distal tibia (*arrows*). Figure 144.4 (sagittal gradient echo [T2*] image) reveals loss of articular cartilage with narrowing of the anterior portion of the joint, as well as prominent foci of low-signal-intensity "blooming" along the anterior and posterior margins of the joint, compatible with hemosiderin (*arrows*).

Differential Diagnosis

Pigmented villonodular synovitis

Teaching Points

▸ Both pigmented villonodular synovitis and chronic or repetitive hemarthroses will result in hemosiderin deposition within the synovium.

▸ Due to its paramagnetic properties, hemosiderin produces low signal intensity on all pulse sequences that is most pronounced on gradient echo images, where it produces prominent susceptibility artifacts (low-signal-intensity "blooming"), as in this case.

▸ The abnormal subchondral changes in the distal tibia would be unusual for pigmented villonodular synovitis and more characteristic of hemophilia.

Management

Treatment of the underlying coagulopathy

Further Readings

Jelbert A, Vaidya S, Fotiadis N. Imaging and staging of haemophilic arthropathy. *Clin Radiol* 2009;64:1119–1128.
Kilkoyne RF, Nuss R. Radiological assessment of haemophilic arthropathy with emphasis on MRI findings. *Haemophilia* 2003;9(Suppl 1):57–63.

History

▶ Young baseball player with elbow pain

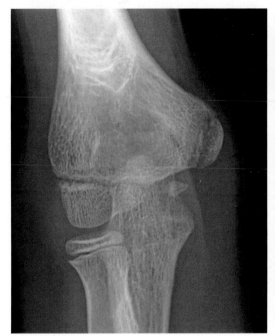

Figure 145.1

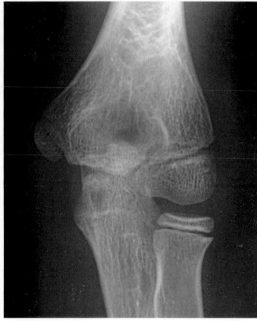

Figure 145.2

Case 145   Medial epicondylar apophysitis ("Little Leaguer's elbow")

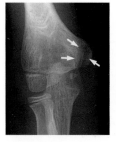

Figure 145.3

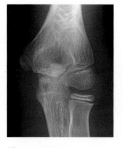

Figure 145.4

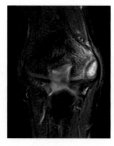

Figure 145.5

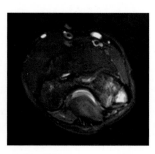

Figure 145.6

Findings

Figure 145.3 (AP view of the right elbow) reveals slight ill definition and apparent widening of the medial epicondylar physis (*arrows*) compared with the normal left elbow (Fig. 145.4). Coronal (Fig. 145.5) and axial (Fig. 145.6) fat-saturated T2-weighted images demonstrate diffuse edema-like signal within the affected apophysis and adjacent humeral metaphysis.

Differential Diagnosis

Salter I fracture

Teaching Points

▶ In the skeletally immature athlete, the apophysis is the weakest link in the bone–tendon–muscle complex and is highly susceptible to acute avulsion or chronic stress injuries.

▶ Within the elbow, the medial epicondylar apophysis is especially vulnerable in young throwers owing to strong valgus forces that occur during the throwing motion which produce tensile forces along the medial aspect of the joint.

▶ Repetitive tensile forces may result in a stress reaction along the medial epicondylar apophysis that is manifested by ingrowth of the physeal cartilage into the metaphysis, resulting in an apparent widening of the physis on radiographs.

▶ MR imaging can diagnose these injuries at an earlier stage than radiographs, given its ability to demonstrate the marrow edema that occurs in areas of abnormal bone stress. It is also helpful for simultaneously assessing the status of the ulnar collateral ligament, which is commonly injured in throwers (though it is more often injured in skeletally mature athletes).

Management

Complete rest from throwing activities for at least 4 to 6 weeks (often longer), followed by a gradual return to activity in conjunction with a reconditioning program

Further Readings

Benjamin HJ, Briner WW. Little League elbow. *Clin J Sport Med* 2005;*15*:37–41.

Index of Cases

Index